WORKOUT PROGRAM FOR BEGINNERS

BIG BICEPS
BIG ABS!

Take Your Body From Flab To Abs in 4 Weeks

DERRICK CASEY

Copyright © 2020 Derrick Casey

All Rights Reserved

Copyright 2020 By Derrick Casey - All rights reserved.

The following book is produced below with the goal of providing information that is as accurate and reliable as possible. Regardless, purchasing this eBook can be seen as consent to the fact that both the publisher and the author of this book are in no way experts on the topics discussed within and that any recommendations or suggestions that are made herein are for entertainment purposes only. Professionals should be consulted as needed prior to undertaking any of the action endorsed herein.

This declaration is deemed fair and valid by both the American Bar Association and the Committee of Publishers Association and is legally binding throughout the United States.

Furthermore, the transmission, duplication or reproduction of any of the following work including specific information will be considered an illegal act irrespective of if it is done electronically or in print. This extends to creating a secondary or tertiary copy of the work or a recorded copy and is only allowed with express written consent from the Publisher. All additional right reserved.

The information in the following pages is broadly considered to be a truthful and accurate account of facts and as such any inattention, use or misuse of the information in question by the reader will render any resulting actions solely under their purview. There are no scenarios in which the publisher or the original author of this work can be in any fashion deemed liable for any hardship or damages that may befall them after undertaking information described herein.

Additionally, the information in the following pages is intended only for informational purposes and should thus be thought of as universal. As befitting its nature, it is presented without assurance regarding its prolonged validity or interim quality. Trademarks that are mentioned are done without written consent and can in no way be considered an endorsement from the trademark holder.

Table of Contents

PART I 8

Introduction 9

Chapter 1: 5 Reasons why most people fail to get bigger 11

Other sources of protein 12

Chapter 2: 10 Rules to increase your muscle mass 16

Chapter 3: How to actually build lean muscles 19

Chapter 4: Tips to keep making gains 28

Chapter 5: Example of a training schedule 29

Weekly training schedule (Monday - Friday) 29

Chest and abs 29

Daily mass gym program 30

Introduction 34

Chapter 1: 5 Reasons why most people fail to get bigger 36

Other sources of protein 37

Chapter 2: 10 Rules to increase your muscle mass 41

Chapter 3: How to actually build lean muscles 44

Chapter 4: Tips to keep making gains 53

Chapter 5: Example of a training schedule 54

Weekly training schedule (Monday - Friday) 54

Chest and abs 54

Daily mass gym program 55

PART II 59

Chapter 1: Setting Yourself Up For Success 60

How Your Diet Affects Your Results 60

Chapter 2: Types of Bodyweight Workouts 64

Chapter 3: Planning a Workout Routine That Works For You 69

Chapter 4: How to Make the Most Out of Your Bodyweight Workouts .. 74

WHAT IS METABOLISM? 79

PHASE 1 84

BREAKFAST 85

CINNAMON APPLE QUINOA 85

LUNCH 86

MASHED CHICKPEA SALAD 86

DINNER 87

SLOW COOKER SPAGHETTI AND MEATBALLS 87

PHASE 2 90

BREAKFAST 91

KOREAN ROLLED OMELETTE 91

LUNCH 92

MARINATED TOFU WITH PEPPERS AND ONIONS 92

DINNER 94

ROAST BEEF AND VEGETABLES 94

PHASE 3 96

BREAKFAST 96

BERRY COBBLER WITH QUINOA 96

LUNCH 98

    ITALIAN TUNA SALAD 98

  DINNER 99

    SHEET PAN STEAK AND VEGGIES...99

DOS AND DON'TS..101

Chapter 1: How to Choose the Right Number of Repetitions 107

Chapter 2: How to Breathe During Exercises...110

Chapter 3: Machines or Free Weights? 112

Chapter 4: Putting it all together. How to program a training cycle 115

Chapter 1: Mastering the Air Fryer..122

AF Buffalo Chicken Wings...141

Country Style Chicken Tenders..142

Beef Roll Ups..147

Yields: Four Servings..148

Chapter 5: Air Fryer Desserts 179

- AF Buffalo Chicken Wings 203

- Beef Roll Ups... 203

Chapter 5: Air Fryer Desserts 205

PART I

Introduction

The world of strength training is growing increasingly chaotic and downloading this book is the first step you can take towards getting a little bit more clarity about it. The first step is also always the easiest, however, which is why the information you find in the following chapters is so important to take to heart as they are not concepts that can be put into action immediately. If you file them away for when they are really needed in the gym, however, then when the time comes to use them, you will be glad you did learn them. What I have discovered after years of strength training, in fact, is that most people think that there is not a theoretical aspect of the exercises they are performing. Instead, knowing it is extremely important to acquire a better form.

To that end, the following chapters will discuss the primary preparedness principals that you will need to consider if you ever hope to realistically be ready to build up your strength over a period of time. Only by having the right knowledge you will be able to lay out a clear plan to get bigger, leaner and stronger.

In this book, you will then learn everything you need to know about strength training and how to take your gains to the next level. The same principles have helped me and other hundreds of people to get the body they desired.

There are plenty of books on this subject on the market, thanks again for choosing this one! Every effort was made to ensure it is full of as much useful information as possible, please enjoy!

Chapter 1: 5 Reasons why most people fail to get bigger

Are you training hard but cannot increase your muscle mass? Read this chapter on the 5 reasons why you are not increasing your muscle mass: you will probably discover that you are making one of these big mistakes. Do not worry, though: understanding the problem is the first step towards solving it.

1. Do you eat enough?

The problem could be easy to solve, do you eat enough? When you embark on a journey into fitness it is can happen to get caught up in exercising and skip on the nutritional aspect. I'm sure you know that 'abs are made in the kitchen'; well, it could not be truer. Eating enough calories (and good ones) is the first step towards getting leaner.

To increase your muscle mass, you have to eat the right amount of the right food, including carbohydrates, proteins, and fats. Your body uses the food you eat to build new muscle tissue after you destroyed the old one in training. In order to do that, it is important to consume enough protein.

Some of the best sources of protein are:

- Chicken
- Fish
- Turkey
- Lean minced meat
- eggs
- meat, broccoli, salmon

Other sources of protein

- Milk flakes
- Greek yogurt
- Quark cheese
- Beans and legumes
- Nuts

A high-protein diet is fundamental to build muscles. Experts and pro bodybuilders have stated, over the years, that consuming 1.2 – 2.0g of protein per kg of weight is a good ratio to keep building lean muscle mass over time. If you are not able to get this amount trough diet alone than food supplements can come handy

2. Do you train hard enough?

If you have been training for a while, but have not made some gains, it could be due to a lack of training. Do you train hard enough? Our body reacts quickly under pressure and if you're not increasing weights over time, then you could run into a stall zone. So do not settle!

Your body is not made to change itself and it is your duty to give it the right stimulus so that it can actually grow. If you want to get faster results, add more intensity to your training.

3. Rest and recovery

Rest is a fundamental aspect when it comes to any fitness routine. Your muscles require rest to grow stronger and that is the reason why so many athletes choose a training routine divided into days. For example, one day they train legs and the day after the arms, making sure that every part of the body receives at least one day of rest (try to train every muscle group at least once a week).

Even sleeping is very important: when we sleep deeply our bodies repair muscle fibres. It is recommended to sleep 8 hours per night, although my advice is to sleep more if you can.

4. Do you drink too much alcohol? Drinking too much alcohol can destroy muscle growth. Alcohol does not contain valuable nutrients but has many calories, 7 per gram to be precise. As a result, it is easy to "drink your calories" without even thinking about it. If you are on a fitness regimen of any kind, it is advisable to avoid alcohol consumption. However, a drink has never killed anybody, just be reasonable.

5. Are you over-training?

Training with high frequency and intensity activates muscle growth. Therefore, it is fundamental to train different days during the week: 4 days of weight training and 1-2 of aerobic activity is advisable. If you begin a program, complete it! Too many times athletes give up or say that a certain workout does not work "for them" (as if this could be a thing), but the key is constancy. It may take a while to see results, do not give up!

Many bodybuilders, like Arnold, have mentioned the famous 'mind and body connection', so try to keep your attention on the muscle you are training while you do the exercises. It is also a question of 'sensations' and how your muscles contract and expand.

Instead of simply doing the training, focus on the exercise and visualize the growth you are generating.

Chapter 2: 10 Rules to increase your muscle mass

It is always challenging to give the 10 rules of anything. However, when it comes to growing muscles, it is important to have some guidance. This is why we give you 10 rules to increase your lean muscle mass for a more defined body.

1. Give space to recovery: it is not true that more is better, especially for the frequency. It is true that you can train only 1 muscle a day and then before you go back to training that muscle should pass 6/8 days, but the organs of "disposal" are always the same and run the risk of overloading. You can make short periods with high frequency, but these must then have periods of supercompensation.
2. You should sleep very well: it is not only the quantity (7/9 hours per night) but the quality of sleep. An excellent component of deep sleep, it is the basic element for recovery and growth. Sleep must be mainly nocturnal, it is well known by those who work for shifts that daytime sleep has different qualities.
3. Eat often: at least 6 times, breakfast, mid-morning, lunch, afternoon, dinner and after dinner; and in any case, use the rule of about 2.5 hours between one meal and another. If you spend many hours between lunch and dinner, introduce two snacks in the afternoon.

4. Eat a balanced diet: with every meal, give space to all the nutrients. Not only proteins and carbohydrates, fats are also great allies, since are hormonal mediators, provide calories and improve recovery.

5. Do not train too long: do not spend too much time working on your endurance, since it does more harm than good to muscle's growth.

6. Think positive: the mind is a great ally for the optimization of metabolic processes; Positivity helps the hormonal systems to overcome the negativity generated by the inevitable obstacles and setbacks of everyday life. It is essential to define the goals (even in the short term) to go to the gym with clear ideas already, aware that you will have an excellent training session.

7. Rely on basic movements: squats, deadlifts, bench, lunges, are the fundamentals; mass is not built by abusing side wings, crosses or arms. Dedicate yourself to these exercises by changing sets, repetitions and recovery times. Then there may be periods in which the complementary serve to unload the joints and give a different kind of intensity.

8. Do not just focus on some muscle groups: first, you have to build a solid foundation, do not do like those beginners who already after 6 months want to focus only on one or two muscles.

9. Use the right supplements: pay attention, do not abuse them, simply select the main ones; good proteins, BCAAs (branched amino acids) or a pool of amino acids, glutamine, creatine, a support for your joints,

HMB. These are already more than enough to support and integrate a diet that must follow the correct guidelines.

10. Choose a motivating gym: well-equipped but with what you really need, lots of dumbbells and barbells, benches and maybe 2 racks for the squat. Usually, in these environments, you can also find training partners to share workouts, goals and discussions. Training in a sterile and "losing" environment is certainly not very motivating and does not establish the spirit necessary to achieve the goals.

The points to be developed would still be many but in reality, with the 10 you have read you are already well on your way to get bigger and leaner. Success is built from the basics, especially when you are just starting out.

Chapter 3: How to actually build lean muscles

It is difficult to build muscle mass, but with constancy you can do it; however, if you want to develop it quickly, you can find some compromises, like accept to gain some fat along with muscle mass and stop some other type of training, such as running, so that the body starts to focus on developing muscles. You also need to eat more by using the right strategies and doing those physical activities that allow you to increase your muscles. Here are some of the key steps to build lean muscles for real.

1. Start with a basic strength training. Most of the exercises that involve the main muscle groups start with a strength training that activates more joints and that allows you to lift a whole greater weight, such as bench presses for the pectorals, those behind the head for the deltoids, the rower with a barbell for the back and the squats for the legs. They are all exercises that allow you to lift heavier weights while still remaining active and keeping enough energy to better stimulate muscle growth.

2. Engaged thoroughly. The key to developing muscle mass is to do high intensity exercises; with a light exercise, even if protracted in time, the

muscles almost never find the right conditions for decomposition and then rebuild. Schedule sessions for 30-45 minutes 3-4 times a week (every other day); it may seem like an easily manageable schedule but remember that during each session you have to engage as intensely as possible. Initially, the muscles may be sore, but over time the routine will become easier.

3. During each training session, only lift the weights that you are able to support by assuming the correct posture. Test your limits to find the right ballast you can lift, doing different repetitions with different dumbbells. You should be able to do 3-4 sets of 8-12 repetitions without feeling the need to put them on the ground; if you are not able, reduce the weights. In general, 6-12 repetitions stimulate the growth of the volume of the muscles, while fewer repetitions favour the increase of the strength at the expense of the size of the same. If you can do 10 or more repetitions without experiencing a burning sensation, you can increase the weight; remember that you do not increase muscle mass until you challenge yourself to the limit.

4. Lift weights explosively. Raise the handlebars quickly but lower them slowly.

5. Keep the correct posture. To develop a precise technique, you have to do each repetition in the right way; beginners must commit to doing only the repetitions that they are able to perform based on the level of resistance. Find your rhythm for each exercise; you do not have to reach muscle failure when you're at the beginning. You should be able to complete the whole movement without getting to bend down or change position; if you cannot, switch to less heavy dumbbells. In most cases, it starts with the arms or legs extended. During the first sets, you should work with a personal trainer who will teach you the correct posture of the various exercises before continuing alone.

6. Toggle the muscle groups. You do not have to keep the same group moving at every set, otherwise, you may get to damage your muscles, so be sure to alternate, so every time you train you can work intensely for an hour on a different muscle group. If you do physical activity three times a week, try doing the exercises as follows:

First session: do exercises for the chest, triceps and biceps;

Second session: concentrate on the legs;

Third session: do abs and chest

7. Be careful not to reach a stall level. If you always do the same exercise repeatedly, you cannot get improvements; you have to increase the weight of the barbell and when you reach a plateau even with this, change exercise. Be aware of progress and see if your muscles do not seem to change, because it may be a sign that you need to make changes in your physical activity routine.

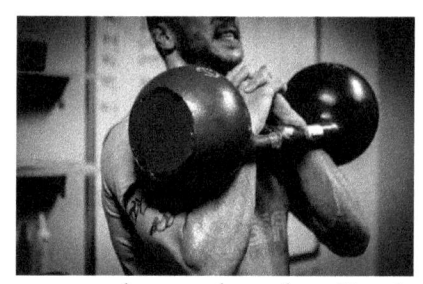

8. Rest between one workout and another. For those who have a rapid metabolism, the rest period is almost as important as the exercise itself. The body needs time to regenerate muscle mass without burning too many calories by doing other activities. Running and other cardio exercises can effectively prevent muscle growth; then take a break between the different sessions. Sleep well at night, so that you feel regenerated for the next session.

9. Create a mind/muscle connection. Some research has found that it can optimize results in the gym. Instead of focusing on your day or the girl next to you, committed to developing a muscle-oriented mindset that helps you achieve your goals. Here's how:

Every time you complete a repetition, visualize the muscle growth you wish to achieve.

If you are lifting with one hand, place the other on the muscle you wish to develop; in this way, you should perceive exactly which muscle fibres are working and you can stay focused on the effort.

Remember that the amount of weight on the bar is not as important as you may think, but it is the effect that weight has on the muscle that allows you to get the volume and strength you are looking for; this process is closely related to the mentality and the goal of your concentration.

10. Eat whole foods rich in calories. You should get the calories from nutritious whole foods, so you have the right energy to quickly accumulate muscle mass. Those rich in sugar, white flour, trans fats and added flavours contain many calories but few nutrients and increase the fat instead of developing the muscle. If you want to develop the muscles

and their definition, you have to opt for a wide variety of whole foods that are part of all the food groups.

11. Eat protein rich in calories, like steak and roast beef, roast chicken (with skin and dark meat), salmon, eggs and pork; proteins are essential when you want to increase muscle mass. Avoid bacon, sausages and other sausages, because they contain additives that are not suitable if you eat it in large quantities.
12. Consume lots of fruit and vegetables of all kinds; these foods provide the essential fiber and nutrients, as well as keeping you well hydrated.
13. Do not neglect whole grains, such as oatmeal, whole wheat, buckwheat and quinoa; avoid white bread, biscuits, muffins, pancakes, waffles and other similar foods.
14. Add legumes and nuts, such as black beans, Pinto, Lima, walnuts, pecans, peanuts and almonds to your diet.
15. Eat more than you think you need. Eat when you're hungry and stop when you feel satisfied? This may seem completely normal, but when you're trying to gain muscle mass quickly, you have to eat more than usual. Add another portion to each meal or even more if you can handle it; the body needs the energy to develop the muscles: it is a simple concept.

To this end, a good breakfast includes a cup of oatmeal, four eggs, two or more slices of grilled ham, an apple, an orange and a banana.

For lunch, you can eat a wholemeal sandwich with chicken, several handfuls of dried fruit, two avocados and a large salad of cabbage and tomatoes.

For dinner, you can consider a large steak or some other source of protein, potatoes, vegetables and double the portions of each dish.

16. Eat at least five meals a day. You must not wait to be hungry before eating again; you have to constantly replenish your body when you are trying to develop muscle mass. It will not be this way forever, so take advantage and enjoy the moment! Eat two more meals in addition to the traditional three (breakfast, lunch and dinner).

17. Take supplements, but do not solely on them. You do not have to think that protein shakes do all the work for you; for your purpose, you need to get the most calories from high-calorie whole foods; Having said that, you can definitely speed up the process by taking certain supplements that have not proven to be harmful to the body.

Creatine is a protein supplement that can increase muscle; usually, it is sold as a powder that is dissolved in water and drunk a few times a day.

Protein shakes are fine when you cannot get enough calories through normal meals.

18. Keep yourself hydrated. Training hard to gain muscle mass can quickly dehydrate you. To cope with this risk, always carry a bottle of water with you wherever you go and drink whenever you are thirsty; in theory, you should drink about 3 litres of fluids a day, but you should drink more, especially before and after training.

Avoid sugary or carbonated drinks, because they do not help your overall fitness and may even take you back when you do strength exercises.

Alcohol is also harmful for your purpose: it dehydrates and leaves a feeling of exhaustion.

19. Try to get to know your body better. Do you know which foods are effective for you and which are not? During this phase of change, pay attention to what happens to your muscles. Each person is different and the food that is not suitable for one person can instead be very useful for another; if you do not notice improvements within a week, make changes and try something else the following week.

20. Sleep more than what you think you should. Sleep is essential to allow muscles to develop; try to sleep at least seven hours a night, although the ideal would be 8-9 hours.

21. Focus only on strength training. You may like to do cardio exercises (sports like running and so on), but these activities require a further effort of the body (muscles and joints) and consume the energy you need to build muscle mass. In general, cardio activities should be included in an exercise routine for general health and well-being, but if you are currently struggling to increase muscle volume quickly, you need to focus on this for a few months, so you can reach your goal.

Chapter 4: Tips to keep making gains

- Always ask a friend for help when doing the most difficult lifting exercises, such as bench press; these are high risk movements and it is always important to have some support to be able to do more repetitions.
- Keep motivation high. Find a friend who's training with you, sign up for a weightlifting fan forum or keep a diary to monitor progress; whatever you choose, the important thing is that you inspire yourself.
- If you currently do not have dumbbells and you've never done weight lifting so far, start with push-ups and chin-ups, which are quite challenging for a beginner.
- Make the push-ups easier: start from the normal position of the push-ups and lower the body very slowly; go down as far as possible without touching the floor with your chest and abs. Later, relieved after resting your knees on the ground and start again. This is an excellent solution when you are not yet strong enough to be able to do traditional push-ups.
- Make sure you stay focused. Take breaks only when you need them and not when you feel tired; it is only in this way that you can develop psychological endurance.

Chapter 5: Example of a training schedule

The frequency of this hypothetical schedule for mass training, provides 4 days of training per week, with about 10-12 repetitions per exercise.

The mass program is a middle ground between heavy weights / high intensity training and volume/pump training. You work on strength, hypertrophy, rotating muscle definition and progression, accustoming the body to weight and intensity of work with a growing load plan, which reaches your ideal combination for mass growth.

It is essential, in fact, to know your body and your own ceilings, to prepare and act upon a successful program.

Weekly training schedule (Monday - Friday)

Chest and abs

Legs

Rest

Shoulders - triceps

Back - biceps

Daily mass gym program

1st day - chest and abs

crossed exercises with dumbbells - flat bench

distances with barbell - flat bench

multipower inclined (or with dumbbells)

cross exercises with cables

crunches (3 sets - 15 repetitions)

abs with elbows in support and knees on the chest (3 sets - 15 repetitions)

2nd Day - legs

45-degree press

squat with barbell

standing calf (3 sets - 15 repetitions)

seated calf (3 sets - 15 repetitions)

leg extension

leg curl

3rd Day - shoulders and deltoids

slow forward exercise with barbell - seated

pull at the bottom with a barbell

lateral raises with dumbbells

push down

French press around the neck with a barbell

bench presses

4th Day - back

pull ups

pullover

pulley

deadlift

curl with dumbbells

curl reverse socket with a barbell

Recovery between the series should be carried out for about 1 minute and a half (1 '30).

The first month these exercises should be performed with at least 3 sets and about 10-12 repetitions, with non-high loads. In case you are not trained enough, you can think of sets of 12-10-8 repetitions, where you start with 12 and perform 8 repetitions in the third set.

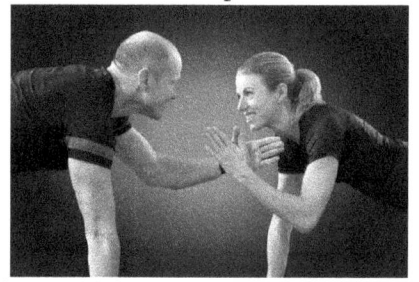

The second month you can go up to 4 sets with 10 repetitions or 12 if the body keeps up with the pace. It will not be easy to get to the twelfth repetition without fatigue and, in this case, you can also think about dropping with weights and get to 12 repetitions with lighter loads.

The third month you have to keep the pace but without progressing too much, with the initials 3 sets of 12 repetitions per exercise.

Introduction

The world of strength training is growing increasingly chaotic and downloading this book is the first step you can take towards getting a little bit more clarity about it. The first step is also always the easiest, however, which is why the information you find in the following chapters is so important to take to heart as they are not concepts that can be put into action immediately. If you file them away for when they are really needed in the gym, however, then when the time comes to use them, you will be glad you did learn them. What I have discovered after years of strength training, in fact, is that most people think that there is not a theoretical aspect of the exercises they are performing. Instead, knowing it is extremely important to acquire a better form.

To that end, the following chapters will discuss the primary preparedness principals that you will need to consider if you ever hope to realistically be ready to build up your strength over a period of time. Only by having the right knowledge you will be able to lay out a clear plan to get bigger, leaner and stronger.

In this book, you will then learn everything you need to know about strength training and how to take your gains to the next level. The same principles have helped me and other hundreds of people to get the body they desired.

There are plenty of books on this subject on the market, thanks again for choosing this one! Every effort was made to ensure it is full of as much useful information as possible, please enjoy!

Chapter 1: 5 Reasons why most people fail to get bigger

Are you training hard but cannot increase your muscle mass? Read this chapter on the 5 reasons why you are not increasing your muscle mass: you will probably discover that you are making one of these big mistakes. Do not worry, though: understanding the problem is the first step towards solving it.

1. Do you eat enough?

The problem could be easy to solve, do you eat enough? When you embark on a journey into fitness it is can happen to get caught up in exercising and skip on the nutritional aspect. I'm sure you know that 'abs are made in the kitchen'; well, it could not be truer. Eating enough calories (and good ones) is the first step towards getting leaner.

To increase your muscle mass, you have to eat the right amount of the right food, including carbohydrates, proteins, and fats. Your body uses the food you eat to build new muscle tissue after you destroyed the old one in training. In order to do that, it is important to consume enough protein.

Some of the best sources of protein are:

- Chicken
- Fish
- Turkey
- Lean minced meat
- eggs
- meat, broccoli, salmon

Other sources of protein

- Milk flakes
- Greek yogurt
- Quark cheese
- Beans and legumes
- Nuts

A high-protein diet is fundamental to build muscles. Experts and pro bodybuilders have stated, over the years, that consuming 1.2 – 2.0g of protein per kg of weight is a good ratio to keep building lean muscle mass over time. If you are not able to get this amount trough diet alone than food supplements can come handy

2. Do you train hard enough?

If you have been training for a while, but have not made some gains, it could be due to a lack of training. Do you train hard enough? Our body reacts quickly under pressure and if you're not increasing weights over time, then you could run into a stall zone. So do not settle!

Your body is not made to change itself and it is your duty to give it the right stimulus so that it can actually grow. If you want to get faster results, add more intensity to your training.

3. Rest and recovery

Rest is a fundamental aspect when it comes to any fitness routine. Your muscles require rest to grow stronger and that is the reason why so many athletes choose a training routine divided into days. For example, one day they train legs and the day after the arms, making sure that every part of the body receives at least one day of rest (try to train every muscle group at least once a week).

Even sleeping is very important: when we sleep deeply our bodies repair muscle fibres. It is recommended to sleep 8 hours per night, although my advice is to sleep more if you can.

4. Do you drink too much alcohol? Drinking too much alcohol can destroy muscle growth. Alcohol does not contain valuable nutrients but has many calories, 7 per gram to be precise. As a result, it is easy to "drink your calories" without even thinking about it. If you are on a fitness regimen of any kind, it is advisable to avoid alcohol consumption. However, a drink has never killed anybody, just be reasonable.

5. Are you over-training?

Training with high frequency and intensity activates muscle growth. Therefore, it is fundamental to train different days during the week: 4 days of weight training and 1-2 of aerobic activity is advisable. If you begin a program, complete it! Too many times athletes give up or say that a certain workout does not work "for them" (as if this could be a thing), but the key is constancy. It may take a while to see results, do not give up!

Many bodybuilders, like Arnold, have mentioned the famous 'mind and body connection', so try to keep your attention on the muscle you are training while you do the exercises. It is also a question of 'sensations' and how your muscles contract and expand.

Instead of simply doing the training, focus on the exercise and visualize the growth you are generating.

Chapter 2: 10 Rules to increase your muscle mass

It is always challenging to give the 10 rules of anything. However, when it comes to growing muscles, it is important to have some guidance. This is why we give you 10 rules to increase your lean muscle mass for a more defined body.

11. Give space to recovery: it is not true that more is better, especially for the frequency. It is true that you can train only 1 muscle a day and then before you go back to training that muscle should pass 6/8 days, but the organs of "disposal" are always the same and run the risk of overloading. You can make short periods with high frequency, but these must then have periods of supercompensation.
12. You should sleep very well: it is not only the quantity (7/9 hours per night) but the quality of sleep. An excellent component of deep sleep, it is the basic element for recovery and growth. Sleep must be mainly nocturnal, it is well known by those who work for shifts that daytime sleep has different qualities.
13. Eat often: at least 6 times, breakfast, mid-morning, lunch, afternoon, dinner and after dinner; and in any case, use the rule of about 2.5 hours between one meal and another. If you spend many hours between lunch and dinner, introduce two snacks in the afternoon.

14. Eat a balanced diet: with every meal, give space to all the nutrients. Not only proteins and carbohydrates, fats are also great allies, since are hormonal mediators, provide calories and improve recovery.

15. Do not train too long: do not spend too much time working on your endurance, since it does more harm than good to muscle's growth.

16. Think positive: the mind is a great ally for the optimization of metabolic processes; Positivity helps the hormonal systems to overcome the negativity generated by the inevitable obstacles and setbacks of everyday life. It is essential to define the goals (even in the short term) to go to the gym with clear ideas already, aware that you will have an excellent training session.

17. Rely on basic movements: squats, deadlifts, bench, lunges, are the fundamentals; mass is not built by abusing side wings, crosses or arms. Dedicate yourself to these exercises by changing sets, repetitions and recovery times. Then there may be periods in which the complementary serve to unload the joints and give a different kind of intensity.

18. Do not just focus on some muscle groups: first, you have to build a solid foundation, do not do like those beginners who already after 6 months want to focus only on one or two muscles.

19. Use the right supplements: pay attention, do not abuse them, simply select the main ones; good proteins, BCAAs (branched amino acids) or a pool of amino acids, glutamine, creatine, a support for your joints,

HMB. These are already more than enough to support and integrate a diet that must follow the correct guidelines.

20. Choose a motivating gym: well-equipped but with what you really need, lots of dumbbells and barbells, benches and maybe 2 racks for the squat. Usually, in these environments, you can also find training partners to share workouts, goals and discussions. Training in a sterile and "losing" environment is certainly not very motivating and does not establish the spirit necessary to achieve the goals.

The points to be developed would still be many but in reality, with the 10 you have read you are already well on your way to get bigger and leaner. Success is built from the basics, especially when you are just starting out.

Chapter 3: How to actually build lean muscles

It is difficult to build muscle mass, but with constancy you can do it; however, if you want to develop it quickly, you can find some compromises, like accept to gain some fat along with muscle mass and stop some other type of training, such as running, so that the body starts to focus on developing muscles. You also need to eat more by using the right strategies and doing those physical activities that allow you to increase your muscles. Here are some of the key steps to build lean muscles for real.

22. Start with a basic strength training. Most of the exercises that involve the main muscle groups start with a strength training that activates more joints and that allows you to lift a whole greater weight, such as bench presses for the pectorals, those behind the head for the deltoids, the rower with a barbell for the back and the squats for the legs. They are all exercises that allow you to lift heavier weights while still remaining active and keeping enough energy to better stimulate muscle growth.

23. Engaged thoroughly. The key to developing muscle mass is to do high intensity exercises; with a light exercise, even if protracted in time, the

muscles almost never find the right conditions for decomposition and then rebuild. Schedule sessions for 30-45 minutes 3-4 times a week (every other day); it may seem like an easily manageable schedule but remember that during each session you have to engage as intensely as possible. Initially, the muscles may be sore, but over time the routine will become easier.

24. During each training session, only lift the weights that you are able to support by assuming the correct posture. Test your limits to find the right ballast you can lift, doing different repetitions with different dumbbells. You should be able to do 3-4 sets of 8-12 repetitions without feeling the need to put them on the ground; if you are not able, reduce the weights. In general, 6-12 repetitions stimulate the growth of the volume of the muscles, while fewer repetitions favour the increase of the strength at the expense of the size of the same. If you can do 10 or more repetitions without experiencing a burning sensation, you can increase the weight; remember that you do not increase muscle mass until you challenge yourself to the limit.

25. Lift weights explosively. Raise the handlebars quickly but lower them slowly.

26. Keep the correct posture. To develop a precise technique, you have to do each repetition in the right way; beginners must commit to doing only the repetitions that they are able to perform based on the level of resistance. Find your rhythm for each exercise; you do not have to reach muscle failure when you're at the beginning. You should be able to complete the whole movement without getting to bend down or change position; if you cannot, switch to less heavy dumbbells. In most cases, it starts with the arms or legs extended. During the first sets, you should work with a personal trainer who will teach you the correct posture of the various exercises before continuing alone.

27. Toggle the muscle groups. You do not have to keep the same group moving at every set, otherwise, you may get to damage your muscles, so be sure to alternate, so every time you train you can work intensely for an hour on a different muscle group. If you do physical activity three times a week, try doing the exercises as follows:

First session: do exercises for the chest, triceps and biceps;

Second session: concentrate on the legs;

Third session: do abs and chest

28. Be careful not to reach a stall level. If you always do the same exercise repeatedly, you cannot get improvements; you have to increase the weight of the barbell and when you reach a plateau even with this, change exercise. Be aware of progress and see if your muscles do not seem to change, because it may be a sign that you need to make changes in your physical activity routine.

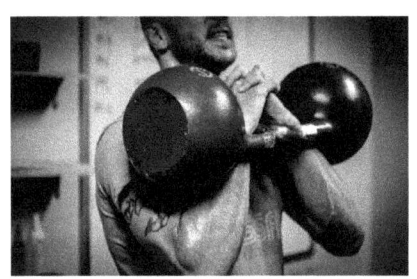

29. Rest between one workout and another. For those who have a rapid metabolism, the rest period is almost as important as the exercise itself. The body needs time to regenerate muscle mass without burning too many calories by doing other activities. Running and other cardio exercises can effectively prevent muscle growth; then take a break between the different sessions. Sleep well at night, so that you feel regenerated for the next session.

30. Create a mind/muscle connection. Some research has found that it can

optimize results in the gym. Instead of focusing on your day or the girl next to you, committed to developing a muscle-oriented mindset that helps you achieve your goals. Here's how:

Every time you complete a repetition, visualize the muscle growth you wish to achieve.

If you are lifting with one hand, place the other on the muscle you wish to develop; in this way, you should perceive exactly which muscle fibres are working and you can stay focused on the effort.

Remember that the amount of weight on the bar is not as important as you may think, but it is the effect that weight has on the muscle that allows you to get the volume and strength you are looking for; this process is closely related to the mentality and the goal of your concentration.

31. Eat whole foods rich in calories. You should get the calories from nutritious whole foods, so you have the right energy to quickly accumulate muscle mass. Those rich in sugar, white flour, trans fats and added flavours contain many calories but few nutrients and increase the fat instead of developing the muscle. If you want to develop the muscles and their definition, you have to opt for a wide variety of whole foods that are part of all the food groups.

32. Eat protein rich in calories, like steak and roast beef, roast chicken (with skin and dark meat), salmon, eggs and pork; proteins are essential when you want to increase muscle mass. Avoid bacon, sausages and other sausages, because they contain additives that are not suitable if you eat it in large quantities.
33. Consume lots of fruit and vegetables of all kinds; these foods provide the essential fiber and nutrients, as well as keeping you well hydrated.
34. Do not neglect whole grains, such as oatmeal, whole wheat, buckwheat and quinoa; avoid white bread, biscuits, muffins, pancakes, waffles and other similar foods.
35. Add legumes and nuts, such as black beans, Pinto, Lima, walnuts, pecans, peanuts and almonds to your diet.
36. Eat more than you think you need. Eat when you're hungry and stop when you feel satisfied? This may seem completely normal, but when you're trying to gain muscle mass quickly, you have to eat more than usual. Add another portion to each meal or even more if you can handle it; the body needs the energy to develop the muscles: it is a simple concept.

To this end, a good breakfast includes a cup of oatmeal, four eggs, two or more slices of grilled ham, an apple, an orange and a banana.

For lunch, you can eat a wholemeal sandwich with chicken, several handfuls of dried fruit, two avocados and a large salad of cabbage and tomatoes.

For dinner, you can consider a large steak or some other source of protein, potatoes, vegetables and double the portions of each dish.

37. Eat at least five meals a day. You must not wait to be hungry before eating again; you have to constantly replenish your body when you are trying to develop muscle mass. It will not be this way forever, so take advantage and enjoy the moment! Eat two more meals in addition to the traditional three (breakfast, lunch and dinner).

38. Take supplements, but do not solely on them. You do not have to think that protein shakes do all the work for you; for your purpose, you need to get the most calories from high-calorie whole foods; Having said that, you can definitely speed up the process by taking certain supplements that have not proven to be harmful to the body.

Creatine is a protein supplement that can increase muscle; usually, it is sold as a powder that is dissolved in water and drunk a few times a day.

Protein shakes are fine when you cannot get enough calories through normal meals.

39. Keep yourself hydrated. Training hard to gain muscle mass can quickly dehydrate you. To cope with this risk, always carry a bottle of water with

you wherever you go and drink whenever you are thirsty; in theory, you should drink about 3 litres of fluids a day, but you should drink more, especially before and after training.

Avoid sugary or carbonated drinks, because they do not help your overall fitness and may even take you back when you do strength exercises.

Alcohol is also harmful for your purpose: it dehydrates and leaves a feeling of exhaustion.

40. Try to get to know your body better. Do you know which foods are effective for you and which are not? During this phase of change, pay attention to what happens to your muscles. Each person is different and the food that is not suitable for one person can instead be very useful for another; if you do not notice improvements within a week, make changes and try something else the following week.

41. Sleep more than what you think you should. Sleep is essential to allow muscles to develop; try to sleep at least seven hours a night, although the ideal would be 8-9 hours.

42. Focus only on strength training. You may like to do cardio exercises (sports like running and so on), but these activities require a further effort of the body (muscles and joints) and consume the energy you need to build muscle mass. In general, cardio activities should be included in an exercise routine for general health and well-being, but if you are currently struggling to increase muscle volume quickly, you need to focus on this for a few months, so you can reach your goal.

Chapter 4: Tips to keep making gains

- Always ask a friend for help when doing the most difficult lifting exercises, such as bench press; these are high risk movements and it is always important to have some support to be able to do more repetitions.
- Keep motivation high. Find a friend who's training with you, sign up for a weightlifting fan forum or keep a diary to monitor progress; whatever you choose, the important thing is that you inspire yourself.
- If you currently do not have dumbbells and you've never done weight lifting so far, start with push-ups and chin-ups, which are quite challenging for a beginner.
- Make the push-ups easier: start from the normal position of the push-ups and lower the body very slowly; go down as far as possible without touching the floor with your chest and abs. Later, relieved after resting your knees on the ground and start again. This is an excellent solution when you are not yet strong enough to be able to do traditional push-ups.
- Make sure you stay focused. Take breaks only when you need them and not when you feel tired; it is only in this way that you can develop psychological endurance.

Chapter 5: Example of a training schedule

The frequency of this hypothetical schedule for mass training, provides 4 days of training per week, with about 10-12 repetitions per exercise.

The mass program is a middle ground between heavy weights / high intensity training and volume/pump training. You work on strength, hypertrophy, rotating muscle definition and progression, accustoming the body to weight and intensity of work with a growing load plan, which reaches your ideal combination for mass growth.

It is essential, in fact, to know your body and your own ceilings, to prepare and act upon a successful program.

Weekly training schedule (Monday - Friday)

Chest and abs

Legs

Rest

Shoulders - triceps

Back - biceps

Daily mass gym program

1st day - chest and abs

crossed exercises with dumbbells - flat bench

distances with barbell - flat bench

multipower inclined (or with dumbbells)

cross exercises with cables

crunches (3 sets - 15 repetitions)

abs with elbows in support and knees on the chest (3 sets - 15 repetitions)

2nd Day - legs

45-degree press

squat with barbell

standing calf (3 sets - 15 repetitions)

seated calf (3 sets - 15 repetitions)

leg extension

leg curl

3rd Day - shoulders and deltoids

slow forward exercise with barbell - seated

pull at the bottom with a barbell

lateral raises with dumbbells

push down

French press around the neck with a barbell

bench presses

4th Day - back

pull ups

pullover

pulley

deadlift

curl with dumbbells

curl reverse socket with a barbell

Recovery between the series should be carried out for about 1 minute and a half (1 '30).

The first month these exercises should be performed with at least 3 sets and about 10-12 repetitions, with non-high loads. In case you are not trained enough, you can think of sets of 12-10-8 repetitions, where you start with 12 and perform 8 repetitions in the third set.

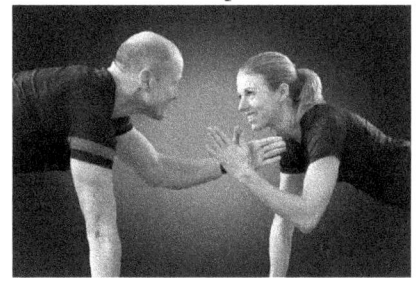

The second month you can go up to 4 sets with 10 repetitions or 12 if the body keeps up with the pace. It will not be easy to get to the twelfth repetition without fatigue and, in this case, you can also think about dropping with weights and get to 12 repetitions with lighter loads.

The third month you have to keep the pace but without progressing too much, with the initials 3 sets of 12 repetitions per exercise.

PART II

Chapter 1: Setting Yourself Up For Success

How Your Diet Affects Your Results

Exercise and diet are equally important factors to building muscle and losing fat. It is generally touted that diet may even play a larger role in the outcome of your fitness. If you are working out hard and not seeing results, make sure that the things you are eating are unprocessed and have high nutrient values—more specifically, work with a nutritionist to find the macronutrient intake levels that are right for the goal you are trying to reach.

Warm Up Before Working Out

To avoid injury, we should take some time before starting our workout to warm up all of our muscle groups. It is generally accepted that warming up before a workout will lead to better performance results and decrease the chance of injuring yourself. Don't forget to stretch after you're done, too! Warming up and cooling down should take no less than 5 minutes, but no more than 15-20 minutes. We don't want all your time spent prepping for your workout or stretching afterward, but they are important components that ensure your body's continued functionality.

Example Warm Up Workouts:

    Complete these exercises for 5-10 minutes

1. Jog, row, or ride a bike at a slow-medium pace
2. Jump rope
3. High knees or butt kicks
4. Walk-out planks
5. Jumping jacks

Important Areas to Stretch:

    Areas are followed by examples

1. Arms: arm circles
2. Legs: walking lunges

3. Glutes: glute bridge
4. Calves: wall lean
5. Back: leg pull

When warming up, we want our heart rate to increase, so make sure that while you are completing these exercises, you are adequately exerting yourself. We want our body to be ready for the more intense activity we are about to take part in. An increase in blood flow, an increase in body temperature, and an increase in breathing rate all build slowly through warming up in preparation. If you need to ask yourself if you are working out vigorously enough, a good test to check is to see if you would be able to keep a conversation going with your friend. If you are working out hard enough, you really shouldn't be able to keep a conversation going.

Who These Workouts Are Best-Suited For

Bodyweight Workouts are best-suited for those who cannot afford a gym membership, don't enjoy the gym atmosphere, or for those who feel like they are too large to jump right into fast-paced routines. Memberships can be expensive depending on where you go, and we don't all have enough money to afford one at certain points in our lives. Many people—women, in particular—feel uncomfortable at the gym or are intimidated by the size of the facility and the variety of equipment. Bodyweight Workouts can be modified for someone of any shape and size and can be completed in the privacy of your own home if you are self-conscious by working out in public.

Benefits of Bodyweight Workouts

These workouts allow you to build muscle, gain strength, and increase your stamina by using nothing other than your body. Able to be completed anywhere and with no equipment, Bodyweight Workouts are fast and effective. The Huffington Post contributor Dave Smith lists the numerous benefits of Bodyweight Workouts:

1. <u>They are efficient</u>: "Research suggests high-output, bodyweight-based exercises such as plyometrics yield awesome fitness gains in very short workout durations. Since there's no equipment involved, bodyweight workouts make it easy to transition quickly from one exercise to the next.

Shorter rest times mean it's easy to boost heart rate and burn some serious calories quickly."
2. <u>There's something for everyone</u>: "Bodyweight exercises are a great choice because they're easily modified to challenge any fitness level. Adding extra repetitions, performing the exercises faster or super-slow, and perfecting form are a few ways to make even the simplest exercise more challenging. And progress is easy to measure since bodyweight exercises offer endless ways to do a little more in each workout."
3. <u>They can improve core strength</u>: "The 'core' is not just the abs. At least 29 muscles make up our core. Many bodyweight movements can be used to engage all of them. These will improve core strength, resulting in better posture and improved athletic performance."
4. <u>Workouts are convenient</u>: "Ask someone why they don't exercise. Chances are they'll answer they have 'no time' or that it's an 'inconvenience.' These common obstacles are eliminated by bodyweight exercises because they allow anyone to squeeze in workouts any time, anywhere. It can be a stress reliever for those who work at home, or it can be a great hotel room workout for people on the road. With bodyweight workouts, 'no time' becomes no excuse."
5. <u>Workouts can be fun and easily mixed up for variety:</u> "It can be easy to get stuck in a workout rut of bench presses, lat pull-downs, and biceps curls. That's why bodyweight training can be so refreshing: There are countless exercise variations that can spice up any workout routine. Working with a variety of exercises not only relieves potential workout boredom, but it can also help break through exercise plateaus to spark further fitness progress."
6. <u>They can provide quick results</u>: "Bodyweight exercises get results partly because they often involve compound movements. Compound exercises such as push-ups, lunges, and chin-ups have been shown to be extremely effective for strength gains and performance improvements."

Creating a Workout Environment

Since these workouts can be complete at home, making sure you have available space to complete exercises is imperative for success. All you really need is a space large enough to spread out a little bit—let's say for example, to complete 10 lunges in a row. While you do not need any equipment, it may be nice to have a yoga mat if you have hard floors like wood or linoleum.

Some prefer a quiet environment to work out or to use a music player to help them focus during their workout. Do whatever puts you in the zone to complete your routine. The point is to try to minimize the space of distractions so you can put in the work to meet your goals.

Summary and Key Points
- Bodyweight Workouts are easy, fast, and are extremely effective for beginners and more seasoned exercisers!
- You can't expect the most comprehensive results without also ensuring your diet falls in line with the changes you want to see on your body!
- Designate a space to complete your workouts in, whether that be your living room or backyard patio.
- Design your space to allow for workout completion depending on space needs and create motivational vibes in the area for inspiration.

Chapter 2: Types of Bodyweight Workouts

Bodyweight workouts can be focused on targeting a specific group of muscles. This chapter will outline bodyweight exercises that target the following areas: arms, legs, chest, back, butt, and abs.

We all have what we call 'problem areas,' and strength training can be the best and fastest way to target those areas on our bodies that we want to be more toned. Bodyweight Workouts use our own weight to create resistance so we can work on building up muscle on whichever body parts need our attention. Here are some examples of workouts from the before-named areas:

Focus: Arms

- **Tricep Dips**
    - This move helps build up your pectorals, triceps, forearms, and shoulder muscles. Push your chest out and using your arms, lower your body until your elbows are at 90 degrees. Push back up. Keep your head and chin up during the process.
- **Crab Walk**
    - Get down into a crab position: hands and feet in line with each other and flat on the ground with your chest facing up not down, knees bent, and hips held several inches off the ground. Walk several spaces forward, and then several spaces back.
- **Narrow-width Pushups**
    - Narrowing your hand placement while completing pushups will engage your core while toning your triceps, pectorals, and shoulders. Start in a pushup position, but instead of your hands lining up with your shoulders, move them in slightly on both sides. Lower your body down, holding yourself up, then push back into the starting position.

Focus: Legs

- **Wall Sit**

- o   Set your back up against a stable wall until your knees form a 90-degree angle with the wall. Your head, shoulders, and upper back should be lying flat against the wall, with your weight evenly distributed between both feet.

- **Jump Squat**
    - o   Standing straight up, keep your arms down by your sides. Squat down normally until your upper thighs are as close to parallel with the floor as they can be. Pressing off with your feet, jump straight up into the air, and as you touch down, go back into the squatting position and start again.

- **Lunges**
    - o   Starting in a standing position, head and chin up, eyes forward, take a step forward with one leg ensuring your knee is above your ankle. You don't want your other knee to touch the ground. Push back up into standing position and step forward with your opposite leg.

Focus: Chest

- **Incline Pushups**
    - o   This form is a great modification for those who may just be beginning and are struggling to do a basic pushup. Find some kind of incline in your workout area: a desk, wall, chair, etc. and stand facing the incline with your feet shoulder width apart and feet 1-2 feet back from the wall. Place your hands on either side of the incline and place them slightly wider than your shoulders. Slowly bend the elbows and lower your body toward the incline, pause and push back up—try not to lock your elbows.

- **Traditional Plank**
    - o   Start off in a pushup position. Instead of lowering yourself and pushing yourself back up, you intend to hold your body in that position. Do not bend your elbows and make sure your feet are not wider than your shoulders. Hold this pose for 10 seconds to begin, and as you begin to master this exercise, work your way up to 30 seconds, 1 minute, etc.

- **Burpees**
  - This move combines several moves into one and can be a killer workout for beginners. Standing straight up, bend down in a position with your hands on the floor supporting your body. Kick back both feet until you are in a plank/pushup position. Quickly jump back on your feet and spring up, raising your hands to the sky. After lowering your arms, start again by bending back down.

Focus: Back

- **Reverse Snow Angel**
  - Instead of lying on your back like you were about to make a snow angel, flip over and lay face down on the ground. Raise your arms and shoulders off the ground slightly, about two inches, and bring your hands down from your sides up past your head. (If you were standing not laying down you would be raising and lowering your arms in an up and down wing-flapping motion.)

- **Superman**
  - Lie face down on the ground with your toes pointing down under your body. Reach your arms out straight to your sides, and raise both your arms and feet in the air while making sure your torso maintains contact with the ground.

- **Good Mornings aka Hip Hinges**
  - Standing up straight with your hands on your hips and your feet shoulder-width apart, bend forward at your waist until your back is parallel to the ground. Engage your core and bring your torso back up in a straight position. It is important to keep your neck in line with your spine while doing this exercise.

Focus: Butt

- **Fire Hydrants**
    - Start in a modified pushup position—the standard pushup position but with knees and hands on the ground instead of feet and hands on the ground. Raise one leg off the ground with your knee bent at a 90-degree angle. This move can also be completed with a straight leg for similar results. If you need inspiration, you want to look like a dog who is just about the use a fire hydrant!

- **Leg Kickbacks**
    - Again, start in a modified pushup position. Try to align your shoulders with your knees. Kick one leg back behind you. Make sure you feel the movement in your hips and glutes, not your lower back. Bring your leg back down and switch sides.

- **Glute Bridges**
    - Lay on the ground, flat on your back with your hands by your sides. Place your feet flat on the floor shoulder-width apart. Use your upper back, upper arms, and core to raise your hips up off the ground toward the sky while keeping your feet and arms on the ground. Slowly lower your hips until they are resting back on the ground.

Focus: Abs

- **Side Planks**
    - Lie down on your side on the floor, and place one elbow underneath you so that you are forming a plank on one side. Keeping your elbow underneath your shoulder, push your lower torso up off of the ground so that the only things touching the ground are your right forearm and the side of your right foot or your left forearm and the side of your left foot. Hold the position for ten seconds, release, and then resume the position.

- **Flutter Kicks**

- o Lie on your back on the floor with your arms down by your sides and your heels flat on the ground. Lift your heels about 6 inches off the ground, and quickly kick your legs up and down. It is easier to complete 10 kicks, rest for 20 seconds, then do another 10 kicks because of how short and quick the kicks are.

- **V-Sit Crunch**
  - o Lay flat on your back on the ground with your arms laying above your head. Lift up your legs like you are about to attempt a crunch, but bring your arms up toward your legs at the same time, creating a 'V.' Lower your arms and legs back into the starting position lying down.

Summary and Key Points
- There are many more exercises within each focus category. The ones listed in this book are just suggestions to get you started.
- If you are confused about how to complete an exercise, YouTube has an excellent variety of step-by-step videos.
- It's a great idea to track your repetitions (reps), so you know you started being able to do 10 pushups and now doing 25!

Chapter 3: Planning a Workout Routine That Works For You

Bodyweight workouts are perfect because it can be completed with only some space and your body: no gym or equipment required! An even better bonus to these exercises is that they are so simple to do that they are easily combined to reap even more benefits in the same amount of time.

What to Include In Your Plan

Important aspects of a workout routine include duration, frequency, intensity, and consistency. The Mayo Clinic suggests adults get in about 150 minutes of moderate exercise a week, or 75 minutes of vigorous activity and at least 2 days of strength training: "Moderate aerobic exercise includes activities such as brisk walking, swimming, and mowing the lawn. Vigorous aerobic exercise includes activities such as running and aerobic dancing. Strength training can include the use of weight machines, your own body weight, resistance tubing, resistance paddles in the water, or activities such as rock climbing."

To break this down for you, you should look at workouts with moderate intensity for 3 days a week for 50 minutes each, or 5 days a week for 30 minutes each. It's up to you to decide when you want to schedule your workouts throughout the week, but making sure you start your Mondays with a workout is always a great way to set up your week for success!

How to Stay Dedicated When Your Resolve Falters

A LifeHacker article written by Alan Henry has some great tips on how to motivate yourself to start your routine and how to stick with your routine. Without consistency, you will never see or keep results!

1. Stop Making Excuses

- Don't be too hard on yourself, we all make mistakes and expect too much from ourselves. Know that failures are an expected part of the journey.
- We all have to start from somewhere—doing something, no matter how small, is better than doing nothing at all!

2. Understand Your Habits
   - "Most people fail in fitness because they never enter a self-sustaining positive feedback loop. To be successful at fitness, it needs to be in the same category of the brain as sleeping, eating, and sex." The key is to find a routine replacement that works for you and gets results for the energy you put into building it into your habits."
   - Starting from zero can cause people to want to give up: "Oftentimes, people are actually lazy because they're out of shape and don't exercise!" It's quite easy for a fit person to tell someone who's having a tough time that they're just lazy, but the reality is that running a mile is much easier for someone who does five every day compared to someone who's been sitting on the couch for most of his life."

3. Find Your "Secret Sauce"
   - "Minimizing and oversimplifying the challenge doesn't help, and while hearing what worked for others can help you figure out things to try, it's almost never going to be exactly what works for you. Look for your own combination of tools, tips, techniques, and advice that will support you and your health and fitness goals."

4. Be Engaged and Stick to Your Plan
   - "Set the bar low and start small. If you're having trouble with working out every day, start with twice or once a week. Whatever it is, start with something you can *definitely* do effortlessly. This is where suggestions like parking on the far end of the lot and taking the stairs come into play."
   - "Whatever you do, make it fun. Whatever you do, enjoy it. Choose something rewarding enough to make you feel good about doing it. If you're having a good time, mistakes feel like learning experiences and challenges to be overcome, not throw-up-your-hands-and-give-up moments."

5. Track Your Victories With Technology
    - "Technology can be a huge benefit to help you see your progress in a way that looking in the mirror won't show you. The goal is to keep that track record, whether it's on a calendar, in an app, or on a website, going unbroken as long as possible. Just remember, quantifying your efforts is just a method to get feedback and track your progress. Your tech should be a means to build better habits, not the habit in itself."

Another great way to keep yourself accountable is by enlisting a friend to work out with you. Even if you don't have the same fitness goals or you don't want to be distracted while you are trying to work out, having someone to be accountable to can really push us to meet our goals. Whether that's a text or a phone call on days you know your friend should be working out, that small reminder may be enough to get them going.

Sample 7-day Routine

After deciding how many days and for how long each day you want to work out, the next step is planning what exercises you will complete in each session. It's not generally recommended that you focus on the same muscle groups two days in a row, although every other day is absolutely fine!

Sunday: Arms

       15 pushups x3

       15 tricep dips x3

       15 lay down pushup x3

       15 walkouts x3

Monday: Legs

       15 jump squats x3

16 X jumps x3

15 lunges x3

24 high knees x3

10 burpees x3

Tuesday: Rest!

Wednesday: Chest

10 second plank x3

15 decline pushups x3

15 mountain climbers x3

15 burpees x3

Thursday: Abs

15 straight leg sit ups x3

20 ab bikes x3

15 straight leg raises x3

20 side twists

Friday: Rest!

Saturday: Back

15 bridges x3

15 back extensions x3

15 opposite arm/leg raises x3

15 bridges x3

Try to complete all four workouts on each day as fast as you can while resting for up to 30 seconds between each move. If you want to up the intensity, slowly increase the repetitions—a good interval is an increase of 5. Another way to make the workout more intense is to complete the workout as a circuit. If you complete a day's workouts as a circuit, ignore the "repeat 3 times." Instead, you would complete, for example, 15 straight leg sit-ups, 20 ab bikes, 15 straight leg raises, and 20 side twists. Rest for 30 seconds! Repeat starting with 15 straight leg sit-ups. Try to not rest for more than 30 seconds. If you need to when you're just beginning, that's completely okay! Complete one circuit and begin working on adding additional circuits to your workouts.

If you already have a workout routine that you regularly complete, try adding in certain strength training exercises between your cardio workout. Again, slowly build up your repetitions but starting small.

Summary and Key Points

- Plan your workouts into your day with your planner or calendar system. Start small and build your way up to working out 3, 4, or 5 days a week!
- Switch up the muscle groups you focus on to make sure that you see full body results.
- The recommended workouts are only a very small example of workouts within each category to get you started. Research muscle groups you want to target and incorporate those goals into your workout plan.

Chapter 4: How to Make the Most Out of Your Bodyweight Workouts

As touched on in the last chapter regarding circuit workouts, High-Intensity Interval Training is a great way to target multiple muscle groups in one workout and burn more calories. We will also touch on tools that can be used to track your workouts and your progress, as well as an important aspect of ending your workout that is sometimes forgotten but still important: stretching!

High-Intensity Interval Training

According to Bodybuilding.com, "these different body compositions point to the fact that not all cardio is created equal, which is why it's important to choose a form of cardio that meets your goals. A recent study compared participants who did steady-state cardio for 30 minutes three times a week to those who did 20 minutes of high-intensity interval training (HIIT) three times per week. Both groups showed similar weight loss, but the HIIT group showed a 2 percent loss in body fat while the steady-state group lost only 0.3 percent. The HIIT group also gained nearly two pounds of muscle, while the steady-state group lost almost a pound."

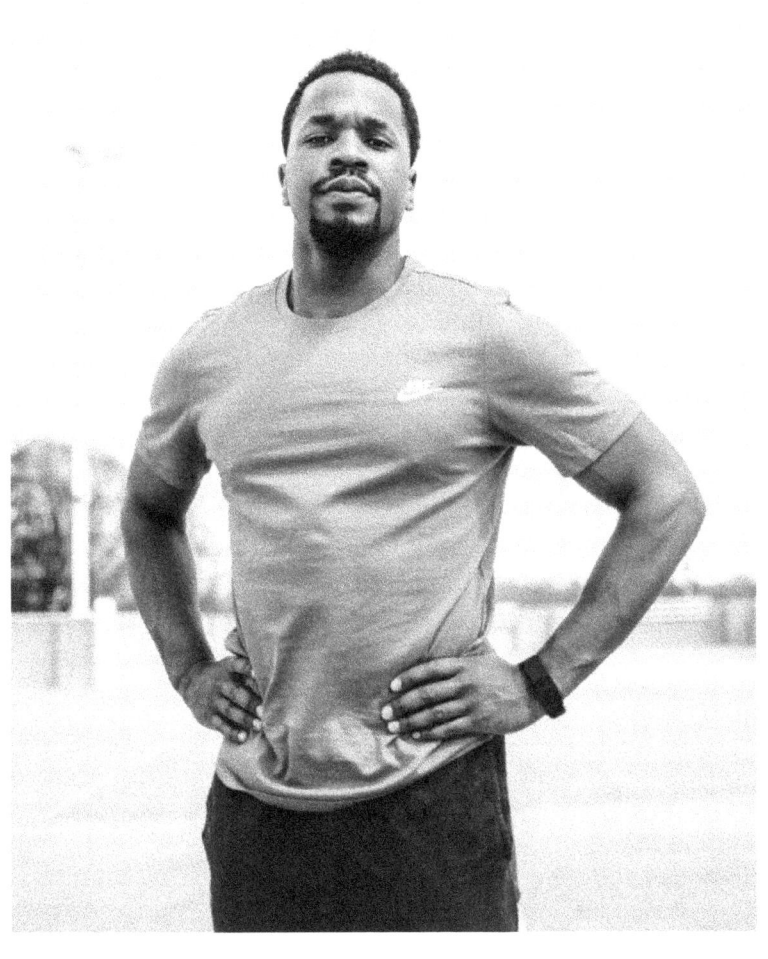

Photo by Autumn Goodman on Unsplash

Progress Can Be Small, But Any Progress is Significant

Tracking your gains is an important part of using body weight workouts. Some people prefer creating their own systems in a notebook or journal, others use electronic devices, and the rest of us prefer to use visual progress indicators.

Writing down when you completed a workout, what exercises you completed, and how many repetitions you completed is a great reminder of your goals and how far you've come on the journey to reach them. Before your next workout, refer back to your last logged workout and see what adjustments you need to make to your workout today to help you be successful.

Technology Can Help Us Keep More Accurate Records

Using a tracking device like a Fitbit watch, hybrid smartwatch, iPhone, or smart shoes, you can track calories burned, distance moved, heart rate, and then have them saved somewhere digitally instead of in a hard copy paper form.

Stretching for Injury Prevention Should Be a Priority

Warming up and then stretching after a workout is an important way to help prevent injuries. Stretch out your arms, legs, back, and any other areas that feel tight.

Key Summary Points

- HIIT workouts are a great way to combine targeting different muscle groups in one workout instead of many.

- Tracking your gains in whichever fashion makes you the most comfortable and that you find the most motivating is highly encouraged!

- Taking 5-15 minutes to stretch after a workout will ease soreness for your workouts in the following days, and will help prevent your muscles from getting injured.

PART III

WHAT IS METABOLISM?

Metabolism is typically used when we are describing different chemical reactions that help to maintain healthy organisms and cells. There are two types of metabolism:

- Anabolism: the synthesis of the compounds that the cell need.
- Catabolism: the breaking down of the molecules to get energy.

Metabolism is closely linked to a person's nutrition and how they use their available nutrients. Bioenergetics tells us how our metabolic or biochemical paths for our cells use energy. Forming energy is a vital component in metabolism.

Good nutrition is the key to metabolism. Metabolism requires nutrients so they can break down to produce energy. This energy is needed to make new nucleic acids, proteins, etc.

Diets need nutrients like sulfur, phosphorus, nitrogen, oxygen, hydrogen, carbon, and 20 other inorganic elements. These elements are received from proteins, lipids, and carbohydrates. Water, minerals, and vitamins are necessary.

Your body gets carbs in three different ways from food: sugar, cellulose, and starch. Sugars and starches form essential sources of energy for us humans.

Body tissues need glucose for everyday activities. Sugars and carbs give off glucose by metabolism or digestion.

Most people's diet is half carbs. These carbs typically come from macaroni, pasta, potatoes, bread, wheat, rice, etc.

The tissue builders of the body are proteins. Proteins are found in every cell of the human body. Proteins help with enzymes that carry out needed reactions, hemoglobin formation to carry the oxygen, functions, cell structure, and many other functions within the body. Proteins are needed to supply nitrogen for DNA, producing energy, and RNA genetic material.

Protein is necessary for nutrition since they have amino acids. The human body can't synthesize eight of these, and they are amino acids that are essential to us.

These amino acids are:

- Threonine
- Valine
- Phenylalanine
- Isoleucine
- Leucine
- Methionine
- Tryptophan
- Lysine

Foods that have the best quality of protein are grains, vegetables, meats, soybeans, milk, and eggs.

Fats are a more condensed form of energy. They make twice the amount of energy as proteins or carbs.

These are the functions of fats:

- Provide a reserve for energy.
- Help to absorb fat soluble vitamins.
- Forms a protection insulation and cushion around vital organs.
- Helps to form a cellular structure.

The fatty acids that are required include unsaturated acids, such as arachidonic, linolenic, and linoleic acids. These are needed in the diet. Cholesterol and saturated fats have been associated with heart disease and arteriosclerosis.

Minerals found in food don't give you energy, but they do play a role in your bodies pathways and are important regulators. There are more than 50 elements that can be found in the body. Only 25 have been deemed essential so far. Deficiency in these could produce specific symptoms.

These are the essential minerals:

- Iodine
- Fluorine
- Magnesium
- Zinc

- Manganese
- Cobalt
- Copper
- Chloride ions
- Potassium
- Sodium
- Iron
- Phosphorus
- Calcium

Vitamins are known as organic compounds that the human body is unable to synthesize by itself, so they need to be found within your diet. These are the most important vitamins in metabolism:

- Pantothenic Acid
- Nicotinic acid or Niacin
- B2 or riboflavin
- Vitamin A

Metabolism's chemical reactions are grouped within your metabolic pathways. This gives the chemicals that come from your nutrition to be changed through several different steps along with another chemical. This is done with a series of enzymes.

Enzymes are important for your metabolism because they give organisms the ability to achieve the reactions that they need for energy. These also work along with the others that release energy. Enzymes are basically catalysts that let these reactions happen efficiently and quickly.

PHASE 1

While on this diet you will rotate the way you eat between three phases:

- Phase One – Monday and Tuesday:
- Phase Two – Wednesday and Thursday:
- Phase Three – Friday, Saturday, and Sunday:
- Repeat this for four weeks.

Every phase focuses on different healthy, whole foods to help reduce your liver stress, calm your adrenal glands, and feed your thyroid. Now, let's look at phase one and some recipes to get you started.

Phase One – low-fat, moderate-protein, high-glycemic

One of the main things that phase one will help you with is by regulating your adrenal glands. The adrenal glands secrete stress hormones, which is only useful when you are in immediate danger. When you aren't in danger, all it will do for you is raise your cortisol level, which causes weight gain.

In phase one, you will eat higher glycemic fruits because they stimulate your pituitary gland, which is your pleasure center. This releases endorphins which will reduce anxiety and stress.

In phase one you will also need to do some cardio, this will help to reduce cortisol levels even more.

BREAKFAST

CINNAMON APPLE QUINOA

Serves: 2

Ingredients:

Honey

2 tsp cinnamon

2 large apples

1 ½ c water

½ c quinoa

Instructions:

Prepare the apples by coring and peeling. Chop the prepared apples into small pieces.

Place the apples, quinoa, and water into a pot. Allow the mixture to come to a boil. Place the lid on the pot and turn the heat down to a simmer. Let cook for 20 to 25 minutes. The apples should be soft, and the quinoa should have absorbed all the water.

Mix in the cinnamon and divide between two bowls.

Drizzle the top with some more cinnamon and honey.

LUNCH

MASHED CHICKPEA SALAD

Serves: 2

Ingredients:

Pepper and salt to your taste

1 ½ tbsp sunflower seeds

½ lemon, juiced

½ tsp garlic, minced

3 tbsp Dijon

2 tbsp cilantro

½ c kale, chopped

¼ c red onion, chopped

1/3 of an apple, chopped

2 celery stalks, chopped

15-oz chickpeas, rinsed and drained

1 carrot, shredded

Instructions:

Shred your carrot in a food processor and place in a large bowl.

Place the chickpeas in the processor and pulse a couple of times until well blended, but a little chunky. If you want, you can just use a potato masher.

Place chickpeas and the rest of the ingredients in the bowl with the carrot. Mix everything together and add pepper and salt to your taste.

DINNER

SLOW COOKER SPAGHETTI AND MEATBALLS

Serves: 6

Ingredients:

Meatballs:

½ tsp pepper

1 tsp salt

½ c breadcrumbs

2 eggs

1 ½ tsp oregano

¼ c parsley, minced

3 minced garlic

½ onion, grated

1 ½ lb lean ground beef

Sauce:

16-oz whole wheat spaghetti drained and cooked

4 basil leaves, sliced

14-oz crushed tomatoes

28-oz crushed tomatoes

½ tsp pepper

½ tsp salt

½ tsp sugar

4-oz tomato paste

1 tsp oregano

1 onion, chopped

3 minced garlic cloves

1 tbsp olive oil

Instructions:

Meatballs:

Your oven should be at 350. Spray a baking sheet with nonstick spray.

Mix the pepper, salt, breadcrumbs, eggs, oregano, parsley, garlic, onion, and beef together.

For the meat mixture into balls. Place them on the baking sheet, evenly spaced.

Bake until they are almost cooked, about 12 to 15 minutes. Transfer your meatballs to your slow cookers and scrape off bits of fat from the bottom of the meatballs.

Sauce:

Place the oil in a pan and heat. Place in the garlic and cook for a few seconds.

Mix in the oregano and onion. Cooking for about three minutes, the onions should be soft.

Stir in the pepper, salt, sugar, and tomato paste and cook another two minutes.

Mix in the basil and crushed tomatoes. Pour the mixture over the meatballs in your cooker.

Cook for five hours at low. Serve the mixture over your cooked spaghetti.

PHASE 2

Phase 2 – low-fat, low-carb, high-veggie, high-protein

Lean proteins provide the ingredients that create amino acids within the body. Alkaline vegetables provide enzymes and phytonutrients that break down the proteins. The amino acids are converted into muscle.

Muscles are insatiable. They need lots of fuel. The more muscle you have, the more fat you are going to burn. Muscle works for you. It burns fat that has been stored as fuel to help melt away stubborn fat. More muscle means higher metabolic rate. Muscle-building is about weight training. You can use your body weight, hand weight, weight machines, or dumbbells.

When you eat lean proteins such as chicken, fish, turkey, bison, and beef, the stomach will start to secrete pepsinogen that converts into the enzyme pepsin. This pepsin will start breaking down the protein into amino acids.

This phase isn't all about eating protein. If you were to eat nothing but protein, your body's pH balance would begin to be far too acidic and you will start to feel ill. To balance out this protein, you will be eating a lot of alkalizing vegetables like collard greens, cucumbers, spinach, kale, broccoli, and cabbage. These vegetables give the body more alkaline thus bringing the body's pH into balance.

The other good things happening in this phase is all the vitamin C that you are consuming is strengthening the adrenal glands, and we know that strong adrenal glands react less to stress.

Iodine and taurine in the vegetables will nourish the thyroid thus prepping it to release the fat-burning hormones that will be coming in the next phase.

BREAKFAST

KOREAN ROLLED OMELETTE

Serves: 1

Ingredients:

Roasted seaweed

2 pinches salt

3 eggs

½ tsp butter

Instructions:

Whisk the eggs together with some salt.

Butter a pan lightly.

Heat the pan and pour in the whisked eggs.

Let them cook until they are almost set, then place a sheet of seaweed on top.

Take a spatula and lift an edge of the egg over the seaweed. Continue to roll the egg over the seaweed. Allow it to cool slightly and then slice into one-inch pieces.

LUNCH

MARINATED TOFU WITH PEPPERS AND ONIONS

Serves: 4

Ingredients:

3 red bell peppers, seeded and sliced

1 red onion, sliced into ¼-inch thick rounds

1 tbsp honey

4 tbsp EVOO, divided

1 lb block medium tofu, sliced into ½-inch slices

Pepper and salt

¾ tsp paprika, divided

3 ½ tsp cumin, divided

¼ c garlic, minced

2/3 c lime juice

¾ c cilantro, chopped

Instructions:

Your oven should be at 450. Place foil onto a baking sheet. Mix ½ teaspoon paprika, 3 teaspoon cumin, garlic, lime juice, and ¼ cup cilantro together. Sprinkle with pepper and salt. Pour half of the marinade into a baggie. Place in the tofu. Seal the bag and shake so everything is coated. Allow to marinate at room temp for ten to fifteen minutes, flip over occasionally.

While that marinates, place the rest of the marinade in your blender. Add in honey, two tablespoons oil, and ¼ cup of cilantro. Mix until smooth, and add in pepper and salt to taste.

Mix the peppers and onion together in a bowl and season with pepper, salt, ¼ teaspoon paprika, ½ teaspoon cumin, and two tablespoons of oil.

Drain the marinade off the tofu. Sprinkle both sides with pepper and salt and place on the prepared baking sheet. Add the vegetables to the baking sheet next to the tofu.

Bake for 20 to 25 minutes, stirring the veggies a couple of times until everything is tender.

Divide the tofu and veggies among plates and top with sauce and the rest of the cilantro.

DINNER

ROAST BEEF AND VEGETABLES

Serves: 6

Ingredients:

1 lb red potatoes, halved

1 bulb fennel, thinly sliced

1 red onion, sliced

Pepper

2 tsp rosemary, chopped

Salt

2 tbsp balsamic vinegar

3 tbsp EVOO

3 lb beef rump roast, trimmed of fat

Instructions:

Your oven should be at 375. Brush the beef with a tablespoon of vinegar and oil. Then season with ½ teaspoon pepper, a teaspoon of rosemary, and two teaspoons of salt. Coat the potatoes, onion, and fennel with the rest of the salt, pepper, rosemary, vinegar, and oil. Place the veggies on the bottom of a nine by thirteen inch pan. Place the roast, fat side up, on the vegetables.

Cook until a thermometer reads 125 degrees Fahrenheit, and 1 ¼ to 1 ½ hours. Place the meat on a cutting board and rest for about ten minutes. Turn your oven up to 450. Stir the veggies and let them cook for another ten minutes. Slice the beef and serve along with the vegetables.

PHASE 3

Phase 3 – low-glycemic fruit, moderate protein, moderate carb, high healthy fat

It sounds counter-intuitive, but healthy fats from raw seeds, olive oil, avocados, and raw nuts will trigger your body to burn the dietary fat and the stored fat. You have kept your fat intake low but flooded your body with nutrients from efficient proteins, alkalizing vegetables, and whole grains. You haven't been eating fats, and your body has been burning the stored fat for energy. You might have noticed that your clothes are fitting somewhat looser, but if your body catches on, and no dietary fats are coming in, it will start to store fat again instead of burning it.

Salmon helps to promote healthy hormone balance in your adrenal and thyroid glands. Other nutrients in healthy fats will start to slow gastric emptying. This helps you feel fuller longer and stimulates the pituitary glands, and hypothalamus releases feel-good hormones and allows your body to feel satisfied and full.

BREAKFAST

BERRY COBBLER WITH QUINOA

Serves: 4

Ingredients:

1 c strawberries, frozen

2 c blackberries, frozen

¼ tsp cinnamon

¼ c almond milk

¼ c maple syrup

1 tsp vanilla

¼ c ground flaxseed

½ c coconut oil

½ c chopped walnuts

½ c quinoa flour

½ c cooked quinoa

1 c dry oats

Instructions:

Your oven should be at 375.

Mix all the ingredients together, except for the berries.

Place the berries in a nine by nine baking dish and then top with the quinoa mixture.

Cook for 35 to 40 minutes or until it has browned. You can also serve with a drizzle of honey and a dollop of Greek yogurt.

LUNCH

ITALIAN TUNA SALAD

Serves: 2

Ingredients:

¼ tsp salt

1 tbsp lemon juice

1 minced garlic clove

¼ c chopped green olives

¼ c red onion, diced

½ sweet yellow pepper, diced

3-oz black olives, sliced

½ c parsley leaves, chopped

1 c diced tomatoes

2 cans Yellowfin Tuna in Olive oil, not drained

Instructions:

Place the tuna into a bowl and break up the pieces. Mix in the rest of the ingredients. You can serve on a bun or a bed of lettuce.

DINNER

SHEET PAN STEAK AND VEGGIES

Serves: 6

Ingredients:

2 lb top sirloin

Pepper and salt

1 tsp thyme

3 minced garlic cloves

2 tbsp olive oil

16-oz broccoli florets

2 lb red potatoes

Instructions:

Your oven should be set to broil. Grease a baking sheet lightly.

Parboil the potatoes for 12 to 15 minutes and drain.

Place the broccoli and potatoes on the baking sheet. Drizzle with pepper, salt, thyme, garlic, and olive oil and toss.

Sprinkle the steak with pepper and salt and place on the baking sheet between the veggies.

Broil the steak until browned, this should take about four to five minutes on each side.

DOS AND DON'TS

Avoid these foods in all phases:

- Fat-free "diet" foods – this includes zero-cal, fat-free, or diet foods
- Artificial sweeteners
- Fruit juices and dried fruit
- Alcohol
- Caffeine – if you have to have coffee, use organic decaffeinated
- Refined sugars
- Dairy
- Corn
- Non-sprouted wheat

Phase 1:

- Meals: 3 meals and 2 fruit snacks
    - Breakfast: fruit and grain, 30 minutes after waking up
    - Fruit snack
    - Lunch: vegetable, fruit, protein, and grain
    - Fruit snack

- - Dinner: vegetable, protein, and grain
- Organic when possible
- All fruits and veggies
- Protein – veggie and animal
  - Lean meat
  - Lean poultry
  - Lean fish
  - Eggs – white only
  - Beans
- Plenty or spices, herbs, broth, and condiments
- Grains
  - Sprouted and whole wheat
- Water
- No fats

Phase 2:

- Meals
  - Breakfast: veggie and protein, 30 minutes after your get up

- - o   Protein snack
  - o   Lunch: veggie and protein
  - o   Protein snack
  - o   Dinner: veggie and protein
- Low-glycemic vegetables
- Lemon and limes
- Animal protein:
  - o   Lean meat
  - o   Lean poultry
  - o   Lean fish
  - o   Shellfish
  - o   Eggs- white only
- No vegetable proteins
- Condiments, spices, herbs, and broth
- No starches or grains
- No fats
- Water

Phase 3:

- Meals
    - Breakfast: veggie, grain, protein, or fat 30 minutes after waking
    - Protein, fat, or veggie snack
    - Lunch: fruit, veggie, protein, or fat
    - Protein, fat, or veggie snack
    - Dinner: starch, grain, veggie, protein, or fat
- All veggies
- Low-glycemic fruits
- Animal and veggie protein
    - Any meat
    - Liver
    - Poultry
    - Fish
    - Shellfish
    - Eggs
    - Beans

- Seeds and nuts
- Non-dairy proteins
- Whole starches and grains
- Condiments, spices, herbs, and broth
- Healthy fats
- Water

PART IV

Chapter 1: How to Choose the Right Number of Repetitions

"How do I choose the number of repetitions and series?"

This is one of the main doubts that assail the neophytes of the gym. I still remember the day I asked my gym instructor about it many years ago. In fact, the first questions that a beginner poses to the instructor in front of a weight machine are typically these: "How many consecutive lifts (or movements) do I have to do with this machines? And for how many times?"

The most precise ones even dare to ask how much time they have to recover from one set to the next one, and so you think you have clarified everything you need to know about a training session at a given weight machine.

The load (i.e., the kg lifted or moved) is generally fixed according to the presumed abilities of the aspiring visitor of the weight room, often without any relation to the first two parameters of repetitions and sets.

There is not a unique answer to these questions since it all depends on the goal. For example, when I first started my training journey, I wanted to get bigger, not stronger. During that period I did a lot of hypertrophy-oriented workouts which worked quite well. When I switched to a more strength-oriented approach, I had to completely rearrange my schedule all over again.

Since the weight training that interests us is not aimed at the practice of bodybuilding—but is framed in the health of those who want to integrate aerobic activities with exercises for the general improvement of strength, elasticity, and flexibility—before defining the number of repetitions and sets, it is necessary to establish the objective to be achieved or what aspect do you want to train for between the following:

- **The resistant force**: the force that the muscle must apply to overcome the fatigue resulting from a prolonged effort.

- **The maximal force**: the maximum force that the muscle can develop with a lifting test (or a limited number of tests). It is also often referred to as a maximal load if referring to a specific exercise in the gym.

- **The fast force:** the maximum force that the muscle can develop to counteract a load in a limited period of time. Referring to time, therefore, more than force we should speak of power which is the ability to develop a force in the unity of time.

- **Muscle hypertrophy**: no reference is made to the type of force that the muscle has to generate, but to its effect on the athlete's body—that is, to maximize the increase in muscle volume. The muscular volume is connected to the developed force, because the greater the cross section of the muscle, the greater the muscle fibers available to make the effort. However, the equation *muscle hypertrophy = greater muscle strength* is not always true because, in addition to having available muscle fibers, the human body must also know how to recruit, and this is influenced by other factors such as the efficiency of the cardio-respiratory system, the ability coordination, etc. This should make those who seek to maximize muscle hypertrophy think only of achieving the highest possible performance.

In a healthy view of strength training, you can leave out the last point because the search for muscle hypertrophy, typical of bodybuilders, is far from our goals. Therefore, we can identify three types of training, each of which corresponds to a type of strength that you want to train and, consequently, to a pattern of repetitions-number of sets-interval between the different series.

Remember that to define a training plan, the following variables must be defined for each exercise (i.e., for each machine in the gym or exercise with weights):

- Repetition: it is the single gesture of weightlifting or athletic gesture that stresses the muscle or a district of the muscles. Generally, in the gym at each repetition, the muscle or muscles lift or move a weight (load).

- Sets: the consecutive number of repetitions. The set can be slow or fast, or the exercise is done slowly, calmly, or quickly, imposing to adhere to a higher rhythm.

- Recovery: the time between one series and the next.

So, you might find a typical 3-row workout of 12 sets of 25 kg with a three-minute recovery. This is a very standard way to get started and the first style of training that I followed when started out.

Chapter 2: How to Breathe During Exercises

One thing that is often overlooked by many gym enthusiasts is how to perform proper breathing during weight exercises. It is a problem that, sooner or later, most of those who attend gyms propose to their instructor.

Breathing, as we know, is an activity that we do involuntarily, but it is also possible to control it trying to adapt the movement of the muscles (or part of the muscles) involved, such as the diaphragm, the ribcage, the shoulders, abdominals to the rhythm that we want to follow.

Consciously, one can control the inhalation phase and the exhalation phase in their overall duration or even suspend breathing by entering apnoea.

A lot of sports and disciplines (yoga, pilates, etc.), give a lot of importance to breathing, while other oriental disciplines even give it a spiritual value.

Even in the exercises that are performed in the gym, including those with weights, breathing has a considerable importance. Unfortunately, there are not many who have clear ideas about it.

Instructors usually advise to:

21. **inhale** in the discharge phase of the action, usually when the weight is being returned to its initial position;

22. **exhale** in the loading phase of the exercise or when there is more effort required.

This usually works well, even if the beginner will at first see this as another constraint which will only confuse him. In reality, it requires a good amount of concentration to force yourself to control breathing in this way and therefore forces the athlete to give complete attention to what he is doing. A lot of times, people look around in the gym while doing an exercise, or—worse—talking to someone. This is something that I have never understood: to me, strength training is a way to become the best version of myself, both physically and mentally, and I do not have time to waste. Focusing on breathing is a good way to think exclusively about the exercise you are performing.

The following is a good general rule to follow:

The most important thing to do is not to hold your breath during the loading phase.

Holding your breath in the loading phase is a big mistake, as it is instinctive to hold your breath during the maximum effort required. Instead, the opposite must be done because this practice can also lead to serious consequences, especially if the effort involves muscles of the upper body.

Holding the breath deliberately blocks the glottis, which then leads to a compression of the veins due to an increase in pressure inside the ribcage. As a result of this compression, the veins can also partially occlude (as if they were strangled by one hand) and this considerably slows the return of venous blood to the heart. As a consequence, the arterial pressure rises, reaching even impressive values such as 300 mmHg (usually 120 mmHg at rest). Moreover, as a consequence of the reduced blood supply to the heart, the outgoing blood also slows down and reduces, which decreases the blood and oxygen supply to the peripheral organs. Less blood and oxygen to the brain could result in dizziness, blurred vision, etc. until you eventually faint. These are side effects well-known by opera singers who practice hyperventilation exercises that, in some parts, are performed in apnoea.

Chapter 3: Machines or Free Weights?

The question is interesting, and the purpose of this chapter is to precisely evaluate the advantages and disadvantages of two possible training solutions for muscle strengthening: the use of gym machines or exercise with the aid of free weights.

From a health point of view, it is clear that the question of the title seems reasonable because, unlike in a bodybuilder, muscle strengthening is seen only as a preparatory to a sport or as a general improvement of the body, and therefore it is not said that the use of gym machines is actually the only possible solution for those who want to make a good upgrade without wanting to reach professional levels of a bodybuilding lover. Before analyzing the two solutions in detail, briefly remember that a muscle can perform an effort in two ways of contraction: eccentric or concentric.

In the first case, the muscle develops the force necessary for the exercise when it is stretching, in the second case when it is being shortened.

Weights and machines are not always equivalent in stimulating a muscle in an eccentric and concentric way. For the purpose of training, eccentric work is the most difficult—to the point that it can also induce pain and muscle damage. It is therefore important that, by deciding which exercises to perform (with the machines or with the weights), it is clear (otherwise you can ask the instructor like I did at the beginning of my journey in the gym) which exercises stimulate the muscles more eccentrically, to introduce them gradually into the plan of training avoiding injuries.

Weight Machines

In the gym, there are usually many weight machines. Generally, except for the multi-function stations, each of them trains a specific muscular district or even a single type of muscle. The effort put in place by the muscles during the execution of the exercise must counteract two physical forces: the weight force and the force due to the friction of the weight that it moves (often along ropes or pulleys).

As a general rule of the mechanics involved in the use of weights, during the eccentric contraction, the friction force is subtracted from that of the weight, while during the concentric contraction this force is added.

Free Weights

They are called free-weight exercises because usually the weights are not tied to ropes or pulleys of the machines, but simply gripped or tied to the body (for example with anklets) and carried out only with the aid of weights such as dumbbells and barbells, which are often seen on sale in supermarkets. Surely, compared to a workout with machines, the one with free weights is easier to put in place. Often, it is not even necessary to attend a gym; a small home space equipped with a mat, a bench (if required by the exercises), a mirror (optional, to control the movements) and, of course, the weights is sufficient enough.

Now let's analyze the advantages and disadvantages of the two solutions, taking into consideration some objective parameters that can assume different importance depending on the individual's objectives, the physical state of departure (sedentary, beginner or advanced athlete), and the expectations placed in a training of this type.

43. Economic aspect: free weight training is certainly cheaper, because, as mentioned, in most cases it is not necessary to get a gym subscription. It can be a good compromise solution to go to the gym for the time necessary to practice the exercises under the guidance of an experienced instructor, and then, once you are sure to perform the correct movements, buy weights and equip yourself with a training-space inside your home. This is what I did, and I would never go back.

44. Versatility: free weights are suitable for multiple exercises and different muscle groups. Think about how many exercises you can do with simple weights to train biceps, triceps, pectorals, etc. In the case of training with weight machines, each machine usually allows a few exercises (if not only one) and this is the practical limit of such a training: you need to choose a gym where there is a sufficient number of machines for the exercises you want to do and where waiting times are not too long. Otherwise, the queues to the machines make the overall workout boring and ineffective.

45. Eccentric and concentric training: weight machines usually lesser stress the eccentric work of the muscle (because of the opposing frictional force) unlike the movement of the body which, in returning to the starting position of the exercise, often performs eccentric work of considerable intensity. Moreover, in the exercises with weights, many antagonistic muscles are trained many times, and in general, they also train the balance and proprioceptive, improving body coordination.

46. Safety and complexity: from the previous point, we can see that weight machines train specific muscle areas, and it is easier to isolate the muscle or muscle district involved. It is also easier to perform the exercise correctly because the movements are constrained by the machines and are easier to learn. With free weights, it is easier to make mistakes, and generally more antagonistic muscles and the spine are stimulated. In addition, with the weights, it is easier to maintain a constant execution speed. For all these reasons, it is generally said that the exercises with the machines are at a lower risk of injury than those with free weights.

Chapter 4: Putting it all together. How to program a training cycle

Now we come to the crucial point: how do I craft a strength training program? The question is very complex. Each strategy will be based on the condition of the subject, so, logically, when we see a disproportionate lack of strength for a muscle group, it will be logical to intervene in this sense. Let's go step by step. The literature on the subject highlights how, for the purposes of muscular hypertrophy and gains in strength, setting a periodized program is the best solution. Before diving deeper into the topic, it is important to note something. You cannot generalize, there is no way to use a unique approach or way of training a particular component. There are countless cases, solutions. So what can be done is to report different models based on different contexts to give not a guide but a concept—something infinitely more precious (and expendable).

Strategy 1. "Basic" Approach. A first approach that we can use is to set up a multifrequency workout by adopting a daily wavy periodization. So we will have two weekly sessions for each muscle district. In the first session we can train the muscle according to a traditional bodybuilding scheme, then longer TUT, intensity techniques, a range of 8-12 repetitions, eccentric, forced, etc. In the second session, we can train ourselves by adopting a progression of strength. So for example, we will train the chest on a flat bench using possibly another complementary exercise (like crosses, chest fly, etc.). A similar approach is at the base of the PHAT (Power Hypertrophy Adaptive Training) method proposed by Norton. Unlike this, however, I find it more sensible to use—in training dedicated to strength—real progressions on exercises without being limited to a 5 × 5 standard type of training.

Strategy 2. Deficient Muscles Approach. Similar to the previous one, the only difference is that a workout in this sense will be done on the deficient muscles while the more developed muscles will be trained in mono-frequency. The increase in weekly volume and stimulus variation will bring an advantage in terms of growth (strength and hypertrophy) that will allow you to "catch up" with respect to the rest of the muscles. This approach can be used on deficient muscles both from a hypertrophy point of view and from a force point of view (i.e., the weakest muscles). This last aspect is particularly important as it can be a valid strategy to intervene where a muscle is placed limiting within the synergy of a gesture. The discourse can also be done from the opposite point of view—that is, to hold the strongest or most developed muscle groups to a multifrequency and to mono-frequency to recover asymmetries (aesthetic or functional).

Strategy 3. The transient phase of reduced volume. Another way to insert a strength training within a bodybuilding program is to provide a period with a high load intensity and a reduced volume. In this case, we always speak of wavy periodization. However, the variations will not be done on a daily basis, but weekly. So, for instance, we will put 2-3 up to 6 weeks of strength training with a reduced volume—less dense workouts but with the intensity of high-load and then return, progressively or not, to traditional bodybuilding sessions, or even to a wavy periodization protocol on a daily basis as described above. Basically, it is a matter of setting a transitional phase aimed at two purposes: Varying the stimulus (Ri) and finding the feeling with the motor scheme.

Strategy 4. Periodization within the session. This is also an interesting approach. It is a matter of inserting, within the session, an exercise on which to set up a forced schedule. In this sense, we could then insert the flat bench into a chest session as a first or second exercise. We will choose a program to improve on strength (since we are already able to exercise the right mastery over the exercise) and set the rest of the session as a traditional bodybuilding session. Obviously, the total volume will decrease as part of the session is occupied by dense work—

not very voluminous but very intense. I find that such a setting fits well with the daily wavy periodization (strategy 1). Basically, by training a multi-frequency muscle, we will set the strength session using an exercise with its progression and the rest of the session in the traditional bodybuilding style. The diversification of work with respect to the second weekly session will be in the TUT (for example) which, in the latter, will be exasperated (e.g., +50'), while in the session of "strength" it will not be too high (e.g., 30').

Split and choice of exercises

A further aspect on which we must dwell is that relative to the decision, within the session, the target muscle groups and the exercises to be used. One of the characteristics of strength programs is that, in most cases, the various muscle groups are subdivided to work only a few each session. This is logical because the work that is required is always of the same type (anaerobic). Okay, as we have seen, it can work on different adaptive components, but in any case, it is always part of the big family of "boosting" work, the same that, in other sports, is alternated with "technical" work. The question that arises is the following: Should we first set the split and then, based on this, choose the type of exercises in which to work the strength or vice versa? Being a powerlifter myself, I would answer "the second," but from a Bodybuilder perspective I would answer "the first." Since this chapter is about strength training, I would say start from this context and, in particular, from the cases mentioned above. Where we want to set a wavy periodization, for all groups or only for some (strategies 1-2-4), then yes, we will have to start from the split. Based on this we will choose the best exercise on which to progress for the strength. So for example, in a push-day, we will choose the Bench Press for the chest, for a pull-day a Bent Over Row, and for a leg-day a Squat.

Let's do an example: Subject 1, Powerlifter, good management of high loads on the various motor schemes. Deficient groups: Arms, Back. Strong groups: Chest, Quadriceps

Split

Day 1 Push Day

Day 2 Pull Day

Day 3 Leg Day

Day 4 Rest

Day 5 Arms

Day 6 Back

Day 7 Glutes

Logically, we will then insert a progression on the Bent-Over Row on day 2 and work the Back with a traditional strength session on day 6. To evaluate a progression on the ground clearance that would be close to a leg workout (even putting it on day 6), we will have the hamstrings on day 7. But training strength, as we have seen, is not just a matter of periodizing and varying the stimulus, but also a question of functionality to the motor schemes to be performed during the sessions.

So let's take another example. Subject 2: Powerlifter, poor activation of the chest on the bench press, poor feeling on the deadlift. Excellent management of the Squat. Deficient groups: Chest-Back-Arms. The goal, in this case, will be to improve the feeling with easier exercises so we will set the split based on the same.

Split

Day 1 Chest and Shoulders

Day 2 Deadlift day

Day 3 Rest

Day 4 Quadriceps and Arms

Day 5 Rest

Day 6 Chest and Back

Day 7 Arms

Finally, in case we go set up a Strength program as a transitory phase (strategy 3), it will be logical to start from the exercises and, based on these, reason on the split.

PART V

Chapter 1: Mastering the Air Fryer

How to Use the Air Fryer

The Air Fryer provides you with a way to eat healthier by providing you healthier ways to prepare your recipes without losing the texture and flavor of your homemade meals and snacks. From *French toast sticks* to *air fried ravioli* or that plateful of *Mozzarella sticks* you have been craving; you will enjoy every morsel as you learn how to prepare the recipes provided in this book.

Useful Guidelines for Recipe Measurement

With so many recipes in circulation for the air fryer (AF) provided greatly due to the Internet; you may begin to notice the many different ways they are written. This is because they travel worldwide and the best ones become viral.

These are some of the conversion tables that will guide you through the process:

Celsius to Fahrenheit

Grams to Cups

Grams to Pounds

Milliliters to Cups

Other abbreviations can include the following:

- Cup = C.
- Tablespoon = Tbsp. = T.
- Teaspoon = tsp. = t.

Going by the 'rule-of-thumb,' a handful should be between 1/3 cup to ½ cup (more or less). You might also hear a smidge or a pinch which is usually ¼ teaspoon or a dollop is usually a heaping tablespoon.

Tips for Using the Air Fryer

Tip #1: Many pre-made packaged food items you already purchase can be cooked using the Air Fryer. Each food may vary with its cooking time. As a guideline, reduce the cooking times by about 70% compared to times in a conventional oven.

Tip #2: While cooking smaller items such as fries or wings; you can make sure they are cooking evenly by shaking the basket several times during the cooking process.

Tip #3: It is important to pat food items dry if you have marinated or soaked them in to help eliminate splattering or excessive smoke.

Tip #4: It is tempting when you are in a rush to attempt to overload the Air fryer. Don't put too much in the cooking basket at one time. You won't receive the best results if the air cannot make the 360° turns that make the cooker so unique.

Tip #5: Allow at least three minutes warm-up time each time you use the fryer so it can reach its correct starting temperature.

Tip #6: When it comes time to clean the cooking basket, loosen any food particles remaining attached to the basket. Soak each of the attachments in a soapy water solution before scrubbing or placing it in the dishwasher.

Tip #7: If you use aluminum foil or parchment paper, leave a one-half-inch space around the bottom edge of the basket.

Tip #8: Cooking sprays are an excellent choice to spray on your food before cooking. You can also spray the mesh of the cooking basket to keep anything from sticking to its surface.

Proof You Should Own an Air Fryer

Benefit #1: It is a beginner's treat. You can locate your favorite recipes and whip up a remarkable meal at home in half of the time. The machine does the hard work for you. All you need to do is program the temperature and times.

Benefit #2: The Fryer Needs Less Oil: It won't be necessary to add oil to the cooker if you have frozen products which are meant for baking. You only need to adjust the timer and cook. All of the excess fat will drip away into a tray beneath the basket.

You can cook whatever meats you enjoy and receive delicious and healthy results. You will understand this once you begin trying out some of these new recipes.

For example; you can cook French fries with a tablespoon of oil versus a vat of oil.

Benefit #3: No Oily Clean Up: You only need to remove the cooking bowl, drip pan, or the cooking basket. It is inside a cover which means you won't have oil vapor deposits on the walls, floors, or countertops.

You can use the dishwasher to clean the movable parts. You can also use a sponge to clean the bits of food that might be stuck to the AF surfaces.

Benefit #4: Purchase Less Oil: It is possible to splurge on the more expensive oils since you only use such a minimal amount.

Benefit #5: Multitasking Features: The Air Fryer is capable of functioning as so many products, whether you need an oven, a hot grill, a toaster, a skillet, or a deep fryer—it is your answer! It can be used for breakfast, lunch, dinner, desserts, and even snacks.

Benefit #6: Safety Functions: The machine will automatically shut down when the cooking time is completed. You will have less burned or overheated food items. The unit will not slip because of the non-slip feet which help eliminate the risk of the machine from falling off of the countertop. The closed cooking system helps prevent burns from hot oil or other foods.

Now that you know how to avoid some of the pitfalls you may have with your new Air Fryer unit; you can begin planning which delicious treat you want to test first!

Chapter 2: Air Fryer Breakfast Recipes

Apple Dumplings

Ingredients

2 Tbsp. raisins

2 small apples (peeled—cored)

1 Tbsp. brown sugar

2 sheets puff pastry

2 Tbsp. melted butter

Instructions

1) Preheat the Air Fryer to 356°F.
2) Mix the sugar and raisins.
3) Place each apple on one of the pastry sheets and fill with the raisins/sugar.
4) Fold the pastry over until the apple and raisins are fully covered.
5) Place them on a piece of foil so they cannot fall through the fryer.
6) Thoroughly brush them with the melted butter.
7) Set the timer for 25 minutes. It is ready when the apples are sold and browned.

Note: Be sure to use very small apples for this yummy treat.

Banana Fritters

Ingredients

8 ripe peeled bananas

3 Tbsp. corn flour

One egg white

3 Tbsp. vegetable oil

¾ cup breadcrumbs

Instructions

1) Preheat the fryer at 356°F.
2) In a skillet using the low heat setting; pour the oil and toss in the breadcrumbs, cooking until golden brown.
3) Use the flour to coat the bananas; dip them into the egg white, and coat them with the bread crumbs.
4) Place the bananas on a single layer of the basket and air fry for eight minutes.
5) Remove and sit on paper towels.

What a delicious treat to be served warm!

Tip: If you have too many breadcrumbs; you can place them in the fridge in an airtight container to use sometime in the future.

French Toast Sticks

Ingredients

2 gently beaten eggs

4 slices of desired bread

2 tablespoons soft margarine or butter

Cinnamon

Salt

Ground cloves

Nutmeg

Garnish: Maple syrup

Instructions

1) Preheat the Air Fryer to 356°F.
2) Whisk the eggs, a shake of nutmeg, cloves, and cinnamon together in a small bowl.
3) Spread butter on both sides of the bread, and cut them into strips.
4) Dredge each of the cuts in the egg mix, and arrange in the fryer. (You will need to make two batches.)
5) Pause the fryer after two minutes, remove the pan, and spray the bread with cooking spray.
6) Flip and spray the other side, returning them to the AF for an additional four minutes, making sure they do not burn.
7) It's ready when it is golden brown; serve them immediately.

Garnish with some maple syrup or whipped cream.

Yields: Two Servings

Bacon and Eggs

Ingredients

4 eggs

12 (1/2-inch thick) slices of bacon

Pepper and salt

1 Tablespoon butter

2 sliced croissants

4 Tablespoons softened butter

BBQ Sauce Ingredients

1 C. ketchup

¼ C. apple cider vinegar

2 Tablespoons each:

- Brown sugar
- Molasses

½ teaspoon each:

- Onion powder
- Mustard powder

1 Tablespoon Worcestershire sauce

½ teaspoon liquid smoke

Instructions

1) Preset the temperature in the Air Fryer to 390°F.
2) On the stovetop, using medium heat—mix the molasses, ketchup, brown sugar, vinegar, onion powder, and mustard power using a small saucepot. Whisk the liquid smoke and Worcestershire sauce into the

mixture to blend thoroughly. Cook until the sauce thickens. Add additional flavoring as desired.

3) Place the bacon on the trays and cook for five minutes. Remove and brush the bacon with the barbecue sauce –flip—and brush the other side—return to the cooker and continue cooking another five minutes.

4) Butter the halved croissant and toast it in the fryer.

5) In the meantime, use a non-stick pan using the med-low setting on the stovetop—melt the butter. Add four eggs to the pan, cooking until the white starts setting—flip and cook about thirty more seconds.

6) Remove from the pan, and enjoy with the bacon and croissant.

Yields: Four Servings

Cheesy Mushroom, Ham, and Egg

Ingredients

3 slices honey shaved ham

1 croissant

4 halved cherry tomatoes

4 small quartered button mushrooms

1 egg

1.8 ounces mozzarella or cheddar cheese

Optional: ½ roughly chopped rosemary sprig

Instructions

1) Lightly grease a baking dish with butter to prevent the mixture from sticking.
2) Preset the Air Fryer to 320°F.
3) Place the ingredients on 2 layers with cheese in the center and top layer.
4) Make a space in the center of the ham and crack the egg.
5) Sprinkle the rosemary and a smidgen of salt and pepper for flavoring over the mixture.
6) Put it into the preheated basket for eight minutes. Take the croissant out of the AF after four minutes to allow more time for the egg to cook.

Yields: One Serving

Scrambled Eggs

Ingredients

2 eggs

Pepper and salt to taste

Instructions

1) Preset the Air Fryer to 284°F for about five minutes.
2) Put the butter in the fryer to melt, and spread it out evenly.
3) Empty the eggs and any other ingredients such as cheese or tomatoes.
4) Open the AF every few minutes to whisk to the desired yellow and fluffy consistency.

Make a scrambled egg sandwich or with toast on the side.

Air Fryer Spinach Frittata

For a fantastic meal good for breakfast, lunch, dinnertime, or anytime; you have found it!

Ingredients

1/3 package (or so) of spinach

1 small minced red onion

Mozzarella cheese

3 eggs

Instructions

1) Preset the Air Fryer at 356°F for at least three minutes.
2) Add oil to a baking pan for one minute.
3) Add the onions and continue cooking for two to three minutes; toss in the spinach and cook three to five minutes additional minutes.
4) Whisk in the eggs, add the seasonings, cheese, and add to the pan.
5) Cook for eight minutes. Season with salt and pepper.

Bacon Wrapped Tater Tots

Ingredients

3 tablespoons sour cream

1 pound sliced bacon (medium)

1 large bag crispy tater tots

4 scallions

½ cup shredded cheddar cheese

Instructions

1) Preheat the Air Fryer to 400°F.
2) Wrap each of the tots in bacon and place them into the fryer basket. Don't overcrowd, keep them in a single layer.
3) Set the AF timer for 8 minutes.
4) When the timer beeps; place the tots on a plate.
5) Serve with the scallions and cheese garnish. Add a dash of sour cream and enjoy.

Yields: Four Servings

Buttermilk Biscuits

These have to be considered for breakfast also because they are so delicious!

Ingredients

½ C. cake flour

¾ tsp. salt

1-¼ C. all-purpose flour

¼ tsp. baking soda

1 teaspoon granulated sugar

½ tsp. baking powder

¾ C. buttermilk

4 Tbsp. unsalted cold butter (cut into cubes) + melt 1 Tbsp.

Optional for Serving:

Honey or preserves

Butter

Note: Additional flour is needed for dusting the counter or cutting board.

Instructions

1) Preheat the Air Fryer to 400°F.
1) Sift together the all-purpose flour, sugar, cake flour, baking soda, and the salt in a medium mixing dish.
2) Use a pastry cutter (or your fingers) to blend the ingredients into pea-sized consistency. Pour in the buttermilk and stir using a rubber spatula (or your hands), and make a dough ball. Try not to over-mix the dough.
3) Sprinkle some flour on the counter surface and begin to press the dough into about a ½-inch thickness. It should be approximately eight inches in diameter.
4) Use a cutter to cut the dough into biscuits; dip the tip of the tip of the cutter with the flour making a swift cut. If you twist the dough; it could prevent it from rising.

5) Place the biscuits in a pan and brush them with the melted butter. Place the dough in the basket of the fryer and set the timer for eight minutes.

Enjoy the finished product with some honey or your favorite preserves, jam, or jelly.

Vegan Mini Bacon Wrapped Burritos

Ingredients

2 servings Tofu Scramble or Vegan Egg

2-3 tablespoons tamari

2 tablespoons cashew butter

1-2 tablespoons water

1-2 tablespoons liquid smoke

4 pieces of rice paper

Vegetable Add-Ins

8 strips roasted red pepper

1/3 cup sweet potato roasted cubes

1 small sautéed tree broccoli

Handful of greens (kale, spinach, etc.)

6-8 stalks of fresh asparagus

Instructions

1) Line the pan used for baking with parchment. Preheat the Air Fryer to 350°F.

2) Whisk the tamari, cashew butter, water, and liquid smoke; set to the side.

3) Prepare the fillings.

4) Hold a rice paper under cool running water—getting both sides wet—just a second. Place on the plate to fill.

5) Start by filling the ingredients –just-off- from the center—leaving the sides of the paper free.

6) Fold in two of the sides as you would when you make a burrito. Seal them and dip each one in the liquid smoke mixture—coating completely.

7) Cook until crispy; usually about eight to ten minutes.

Yields: Four Mini Burritos

Chapter 3: Lunch Recipes

Grilled Cheese Sandwich

Ingredients

½ Cup sharp cheddar cheese

4 Slices white bread or brioche

¼ Cup melted butter

Instructions

1) Pre-set the Air Fryer temperature to 360°F.
2) Spread butter on each side of all of the bread slices, and put the cheese on two of them; putting them together. Cook until browned, about five

to seven minutes.

Yields: Serves Two

Cheeseburger Mini Sliders

Ingredients

6 Slices cheddar cheese

1 Pound ground beef

6 Dinner Rolls

Black pepper and Salt

Instructions

1) Pre-set the heat on the Air Fryer to 390°F.

2) Form 6 (2 ½-ounce) patties and flavor with the pepper and salt

3) Place the burgers on the AF basket for ten minutes.

4) Take them from the cooker and add the cheese; returning to the Air

Fryer for an additional minute until the cheese melts. Yummy!

Yields: Serves Three

Pigs In A Blanket

Ingredients

1 (Eight-ounce) Can crescent rolls

1 (Twelve-ounce) Package cocktail franks

Instructions

1) Preheat the Air Fryer to 330°F.

2) Drain the franks and thoroughly dry them using two paper towels.

3) Slice the dough into strips of about 1 ½ inches x 1-inch (rectangular).

4) Roll the dough around the franks leaving the ends open. Put them in the freezer to firm-up for about five minutes.

5) Take them out, and put them in the AF for six to eight minutes. Adjust the temperature to 390°F, and continue to cook for approximately three minutes.

Yields: Serves Four

Chicken

AF Chicken 'Fried'

Ingredients

2 chicken thighs (skinless)

3 sprigs fresh parsley

Garlic powder (to dust the thighs)

Salt and black pepper if desired

½ a lemon

Chili flakes as you like

1 to 2 sprigs fresh rosemary

Instructions

1) Rinse the thighs. Drain them between two paper towels. (Discard the towels and wash your hands.)
2) Clean the rosemary sprigs and remove the stems. Chop or mince the parsley.
3) *For the Marinate*: Combine the salt and pepper, garlic powder, rosemary leaves, parsley, chili flakes, and lemon juice. Add the thighs and marinate overnight in the refrigerator.
4) *Preheat the Air Fryer*: Set the AF to 356°F.
5) Grill for 12 minutes.

Note: Times may vary depending on the thickness/size of the thighs.

AF Buffalo Chicken Wings

Ingredients

5 chicken wings (about 14 ounces)

½ teaspoon garlic powder (optional)

2 teaspoons cayenne pepper

2 tablespoons red hot sauce

1 tablespoon (15 grams) melted butter

Fresh black pepper and salt to taste

Instructions

1) Preheat the Air Fryer at 356°F.
2) Cut the wings into three sections (the end tip, mid joint, and drumstick). Pat each one thoroughly dry using a paper towel. Wash your wash right away to prevent cross contamination.
3) Combine a dash of pepper and salt, the garlic powder, and cayenne pepper in a plate. Lightly coat the wings with the powder.
4) Place the chicken on the wire rack and back for 15 minutes; turning once at 7 minutes.

5) Combine the hot sauce, and melted butter in a dish to garnish the baked chicken when it is time to be served.

Notes: Save and freeze the end tip for preparing chicken stock.

You can increase the cayenne pepper if you want it hotter.

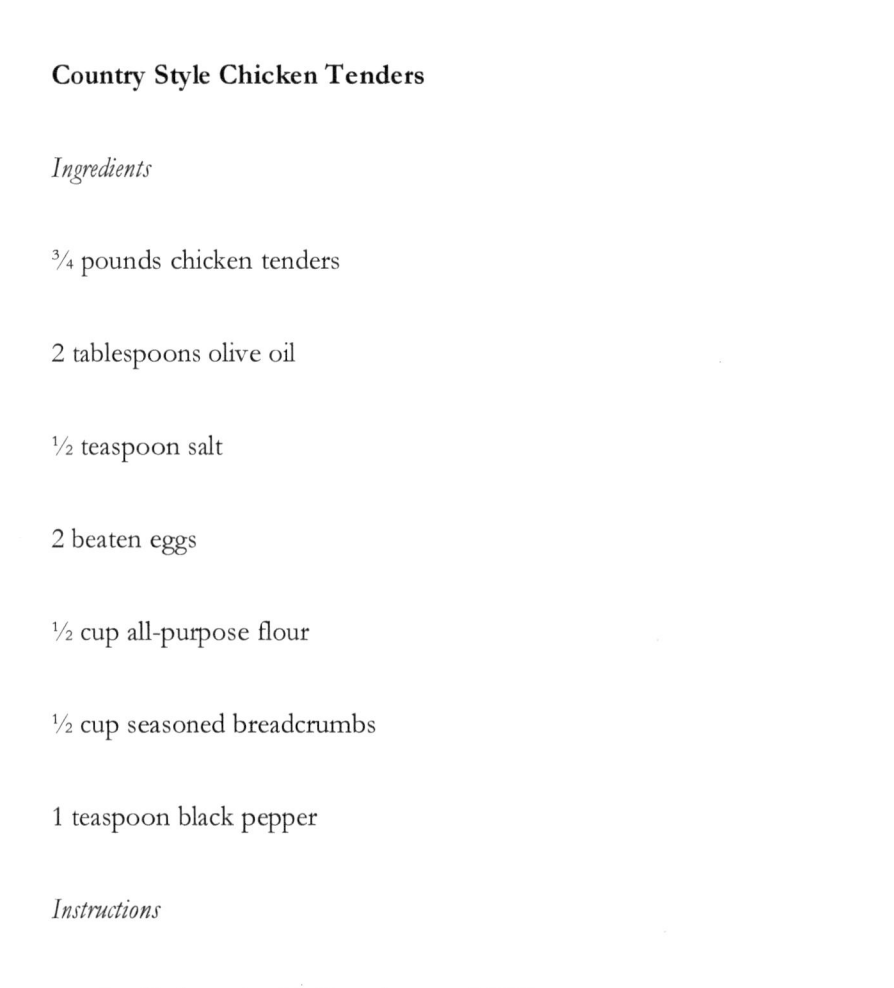

Country Style Chicken Tenders

Ingredients

¾ pounds chicken tenders

2 tablespoons olive oil

½ teaspoon salt

2 beaten eggs

½ cup all-purpose flour

½ cup seasoned breadcrumbs

1 teaspoon black pepper

Instructions

1) Preheat the Air Fryer heat to 330°F.
2) Set up three separate dishes for the flour, eggs, and breadcrumbs.

3) Blend the salt, pepper and bread crumbs. Pour in the oil with the breadcrumbs and mix. Put the chicken tenders into the flour, and the eggs. Coat evenly with the breadcrumbs. Shake the excess off before placing in the Air Fryer basket.

4) Cook for ten minutes at 330°F and increase to 390°F for five minutes or until they are a nice golden brown.

Chinese Chicken Wings

Ingredients

4 chicken wings

Salt and pepper to taste

1 tablespoon each:

- Chinese spice
- Mixed spice
- Soy sauce

Instructions

Preheat the AF to 180°C/356°F.

1) Add the seasonings into a large mixing container—stirring thoroughly.
2) Blend the seasonings over the chicken wings until each piece is covered.

3) Put some aluminum foil on the base of the AF (similar to how you cover a baking tray), and add the chicken sprinkling any remnants over the chicken. Cook for 15 minutes.

4) Flip the chicken and cook another 15 minutes at 200C/392F.

Yields: Two Servings

Chicken Pot Pie

Ingredients

6 chicken tenders

2 potatoes

1 ½ cups condensed cream of celery soup

¾ cup heavy cream

1 thyme sprig

1 whole dried bay leaf

5 refrigerated buttermilk biscuits (dough)

1 tablespoon milk

1 egg yolk

Instructions

1) Preheat the Air Fryer at 320°F.

2) Peel and dice the potatoes.

3) Mix all of the ingredients in a pan except for the milk, egg yolk, and biscuits. Bring them to a boil using medium heat.

4) Empty the mixture into the baking tin and use some aluminum foil to cover the top. Place the pan into the fry basket. Set the timer for 15 minutes.

5) Meanwhile, after the pie completes the cycle make an egg wash with the milk and egg yolk. Place the biscuits on the baking pan and brush with the egg wash mixture.

6) Set the timer to 300°F for an additional ten minutes.

7) Your pie is ready when the biscuits are golden brown.

Yields: Four Servings

Tarragon Chicken

Ingredients

1 skinless and boneless chicken breast

⅛ Teaspoon fresh ground black pepper

½ Teaspoon unsalted butter

⅛ Teaspoon kosher salt

¼ Cup dried tarragon

Instructions

1) Pre-set the cooker to 390°F.

2) Cut a piece of heavy-duty aluminum foil—approximately 12 x 12 or

you can double a regular strength one and fold in half. Put the chicken on it.

3) Place the butter and tarragon on top of the chicken and flavor with pepper and salt—loosely wrapping the chicken for minimal airflow.

4) Cook for 12 minutes in the Air Fryer basket, remove the meal from the wrapper and enjoy.

Beef

Beef Roll Ups

Ingredients

6 slices provolone cheese

2 pounds beef flank steak

3 tablespoons pesto

¾ cup fresh baby spinach

1 teaspoon each sea salt and ground black pepper

3-ounces roasted red bell peppers

Instructions

1) Preheat the Air Fryer cooker to 400°F.
2) Open the steak up and add the butter and pesto evenly on the meat.
3) Layer in the spinach, peppers, and cheese about three-quarters the way down through the meat.
4) Roll the mixture and secure it with toothpicks or skewers.
5) Set the timer for 14 minutes; flipping the beef halfway through the cooking process.
6) Let the meat rest for a minimum of ten minutes before attempting to cut and serve the tasty delight.

Yields: Four Servings

Air Fried Ravioli

Ingredients

1 package meat or cheese ravioli

1 jar Marinara sauce

2 C. breadcrumbs (Italian-style)

1 C. buttermilk

¼ C. Parmesan cheese

Olive oil

Note: Purchase the sauce and ravioli ready-made.

Instructions

1) Preheat the Air Fryer to 200°F.
2) Empty the buttermilk into a container and dip the ravioli.
3) Put a spoonful of oil to the breadcrumbs. Coat the ravioli with the crumbs.
4) Add the ravioli into the AF on baking paper for around five minutes.

Roasted Veggie Pasta Salad

Ingredients

4 ounces brown mushrooms

1 red onion

1 yellow squash

1 zucchini

1 each bell peppers

- Red
- Green
- Orange

Pinch of Fresh ground pepper and salt

1 teaspoon Italian seasoning

1 cup grape tomatoes

½ cup pitted Kalamata olives

1 pound cooked Rigatoni or Penne Rigate

¼ cup olive oil

2 tablespoons fresh chopped basil

3 tablespoons balsamic vinegar

Instructions

1) Cut the squash and zucchini into half-moons. Cut the peppers into large chunks and slice the red onion. Slice the tomatoes and olives in half.
2) Preheat the Air Fryer to 380°F.
3) Put the mushrooms, peppers, red onion, squash, and zucchini in a large container.
4) Drizzle with some of the oil—tossing well. Sprinkle in the pepper, salt, and Italian seasoning.

5) Place in the Air Fryer until the veggies are soft (not mushy), usually about for 12 to 15 minutes. For even roasting; shake the basket about halfway through the cooking cycle.

6) Combine the roasted veggies, olives, cooked pasta, and tomatoes, in a large container; mix well. Add the vinegar, and toss. (Use as little oil as possible, just enough to coat the vegetables.)

7) Keep it refrigerated until ready to serve—adding the fresh basil for last.

Yields: Six to Eight Servings

Chapter 4: Air Fryer Dinner Recipes

Chicken and Turkey Recipes

Lemon Rosemary Chicken

Ingredients

1 pound chicken (350 g)

For the Marinate:

1 tablespoon soy sauce

½ tablespoon olive oil

1 teaspoon minced ginger

For the Sauce:

3 tablespoons brown sugar

1 tablespoon oyster sauce

½ wedge-cut lemon in skins

Optional: 15 g (0.5 ounces) fresh rosemary

Instructions

1) Leave the skin on the rosemary and chop.
2) Blend all of the marinade components.. Pour over the chicken. Let them cool off in the fridge for about thirty minutes.
3) Place the marinade and chicken in a baking dish, and bake for six minutes in the AF at 392°F.

4) Blend all of the sauce ingredients (minus the lemon).

5) Pour the mixture over the chicken when it is about half baked.

6) Place the lemon wedges in the pan evenly and squeeze so the zest will heighten the flavor of the chicken. Continue baking for an additional 13 minutes turning to ensure all of the pieces are browned evenly.

Note: You can omit the rosemary.

Jamaican Chicken Meatballs

Ingredients

1 large peeled and diced onion

2 large chicken breasts

1 teaspoon chili powder

2 tablespoons honey

Pepper and salt to taste

3 tablespoons soy sauce

1 tablespoon each:

- Dry mustard
- Cumin
- Thyme
- Basil

Optional: 2 teaspoons Jerk Paste

Instructions

1) Using a blender—mince the chicken; add the onion and mince; mix well. Toss in the Jamaican seasonings and blend again. Make ten medium balls.
2) Place on the baking mat in the AF and cook at 356°F or 180°C.
3) Put them on a stick when done cooking and some use of the extra sauce over the meatballs.
4) Add several herbs on the top, serve, and enjoy.

Yields: Ten Servings

Note: In case you are not aware; jerk paste is a combination of brown spices, ginger, peppers, and thyme.

Roast Turkey Breast

Ingredients

1 tablespoon ground black pepper

8 pounds bone-in turkey breast

2 tablespoon each:

- Olive oil
- Sea salt

Instructions

1) Preheat the Air Fryer on 360°F.
2) Rub the turkey with olive oil and flavor with the seasonings.
3) Put the turkey in the preheated basket for 20 minutes.

4) When done, flip it over and adjust the cooking time for another 20 minutes (also at 360°F).

5) The breast of turkey is done when it registers 165°F when thermometer tested.

6) Allow the meat rest a minimum of 20 minutes before serving.

Spicy Rolled Meat

Ingredients

1 (1.6 pounds/500 g) turkey breast fillet

½ tsp. chili powder

1 ½ tsp. ground cumin

1 crushed garlic clove

1 tsp. cinnamon

2 Tbsp. olive oil

1 small finely chopped onion

2 Tbsp. flat-leafed parsley (finely chopped)

Needed: Rolled meat String

Instructions

1) Preset the heat on the Air Fryer at 356°F/180°C.

2) Put the meat onto a cutting board with the short end facing you. Cut the full length of the fillet. Stop cutting about (2 cm, 13/16inches) from the edge and about 1/3 of the way from the top. Fold this section open and cut it again from this side and open the meat.

3) Combine the cinnamon, chili powder, 1 teaspoon of salt, pepper, and cumin in a mixing container in a small mixing container. Pour in the oil.

4) Spoon one tablespoon of the mixture into a small dish and add the parsley and onion.

5) Use the mixture to coat the meat.

6) Tie it starting at 1 ¼-inch intervals.

7) Rub the outside with the herbal mixture for about 40 minutes or until nicely browned.

Yields: Four Servings

Fish and Seafood

Salmon Patties

Ingredients

1 salmon portion (about 7 ounces)

3 large russet potatoes (about 14 ounces)

1/3 cup frozen veggies (parboiled & drained)

2 dill sprinkles

Dash of salt and pepper

1 egg

Coating: breadcrumbs

Olive oil spray

Instructions

1) Set the Air Fryer to 356°F.

2) Peel and chop the potatoes into small bits and boil for about ten minutes.

3) Mash and place in the fridge to chill.

4) Grill the salmon for five minutes, flake it apart and set it to the side.

5) Combine all of the ingredients and shape into patties.

6) Evenly coat with the breadcrumbs, and spray them with a bit of olive spray.

7) Place in the Air Fryer for ten to twelve minutes.

Yields: Six to Eight Patties

Dill Salmon

Ingredients for the Salmon

4 (6-ounce pieces) or 1 ½ pounds salmon

1 Pinch of salt

2 Teaspoons olive oil

Ingredients for the Dill Sauce

½ cup each:

- Sour cream
- Non-fat Greek yogurt
- 2 (finely chopped) tablespoons dill
- 1 Pinch of salt

Instructions

1) Preheat the AF to 270°F.

2) Slice the salmon into the four portions, and drizzle with half of the oil (1 teaspoon). Flavor with a pinch of salt and add to the basket for about 20 to 23 minutes.

3) *Make the Sauce*: Blend the sour cream, yogurt, salt, and dill in a mixing container. Pour the sauce over the cooked salmon as a garnish with a pinch of the chopped dill.

Yields: Serves Four

Halibut Steak With a Teriyaki Glazed Sauce

Ingredients

1 Lb. halibut steak

Ingredients for the Marinade

½ cup mirin (Japanese cooking wine)

2/3 cup low-sodium soy sauce

¼ cup sugar

¼ cup orange juice

2 tablespoons lime juice

¼ teaspoon each:

- Ground ginger

- Crushed red pepper flakes

1 smashed garlic clove

Instructions

1) Preheat the Air Fryer to 390°F.
2) Combine all of the marinade ingredients in a saucepan, bring it to a boil and reduce to medium heat; cool.
3) Pour half of the marinade in a resealable plastic bag with the halibut. Chill in the fridge for thirty minutes.
4) Cook the halibut for ten to twelve minutes. Brush some of the remaining glaze over the steak.
5) Serve over top a bed of rice. Add a little basil or mint for some extra jazz.

Yields: Serves Three

Cajun Shrimp

Ingredients

1 tablespoon olive oil

½ teaspoon Old Bay seasoning

16 to 20 (1 ¼ pounds) tiger shrimp

¼ teaspoon each:

- smoked paprika
- cayenne pepper

1 pinch of salt

Instructions

1) Preheat the Air Fryer to 390°F.
2) Mix all of the ingredients and coat the shrimp with the oil and spices.
3) Place the shrimp into the basket and cook for five minutes.
4) Complement the meal with some rice and place the shrimp on top for a tasty luncheon treat.

Coconut Shrimp

Ingredients

12 Large raw shrimp

1 tablespoon cornstarch

½ tablespoon oil

1 Cup each:

- Raw egg whites
- Unsweetened dried coconut

- White all-purpose flour

- Panko

Instructions

1) Drain the shrimp on towels
2) Preheat the AF to 350°F.
3) Combine the coconut and panko in a container and set it to the side; blend the cornstarch and oil in another dish.
4) Put the egg whites into another container, and a third one for the coconut mix.
5) Cover each shrimp in the cornstarch mix, the egg whites, and lastly the coconut mixture.
6) Cook for ten minutes; flipping them after five minutes for even cooking.

Yields: Three Servings

Beef

Rib Steak

Ingredients

1 Tablespoon of steak rub

2 pounds rib steaks

1 Tablespoon of olive oil

Instructions

1) Before it is time to cook; preheat the Air Fryer to 400°F.

2) Flavor the meat on all areas with the oil and rub.

3) Put it in the basket for 14 minutes, flipping after seven minutes.

4) Let it rest for at least ten minutes before you slice and serve.

Yields: Two Servings

Stromboli

Ingredients

1 (12-ounce) refrigerated pizza crust

¾ cup Mozzarella shredded cheese

3 cups shredded cheddar cheese

1 tablespoon milk

1 egg yolk

1/3 pound sliced cooked ham

3 ounces roasted red bell peppers

Instructions

1) Preheat the Air Fryer at 360°F.

2) Roll the dough until it is around ¼-inch thick.

3) Layer in the peppers, ham, and cheese on one side of the dough and fold to seal.

4) Combine the milk and eggs to brush the dough.

5) Put the Stromboli in the basket and set the timer for 15 minutes. Check it every five minutes or so—flip the Stromboli to the other side for thorough cooking.

Yields: Four Servings

Roasted Rack of Lamb with a Macadamia Crust

Ingredients

1 clove of garlic

1 Tbsp. olive oil

Pepper and salt

1 ¾ pounds - rack of lamb

Ingredients for the Crust

3 ounces Macadamia nuts (unsalted)

1 tablespoon each

- Fresh rosemary
- Breadcrumbs

1 egg

Instructions

1) Preheat the Air Fryer to 220°F.
2) Chop the garlic clove into tiny bits. Make the garlic oil by combining the garlic and oil. Brush the lamb and flavor with salt and pepper.
3) Chop the nuts to a fine consistency in a bowl and blend in the rosemary and breadcrumbs. Beat/whip the egg in another dish.

4) Dredge the meat through the egg mixture and coat with the macadamia crust topping.

5) Place the rack of lamb in the Air Fryer basket—setting the timer for 30 minutes.

6) After the time is lapsed; raise the heat to 390°F—setting the time for an additional five minutes.

7) Take the meat from the fryer and let it rest for about ten minutes covered with some aluminum foil.

Substitutes: You can use cashews, hazelnuts, pistachios, or almonds if you would like a change of pace.

Crispy Tofu

Ingredients

2 tsp. toasted sesame oil

2 Tbsp. soy sauce

1 tsp. seasoned rice vinegar

1 block firm pressed tofu

1 tablespoon cornstarch or potato starch

Instructions

1) Cut the tofu into 1-inch cubes. Preheat the Air Fryer to 370°F.

2) In a shallow dish, mix the vinegar, soy sauce, oil, and tofu. Let the combination marinate for 15 to 30 minutes. Toss the marinated product with the cornstarch and add it to the AF basket.

3) Cook for 20 minutes, shaking the basket halfway through the cooking cycle.

Yields: Four Servings

Sides

Bread Rolls with Potato Stuffing

Ingredients

8 slices bread (white part only)

5 large potatoes

1 small bunch finely chopped coriander

2 seeded and finely chopped green chilies

½ teaspoon turmeric

2 curry leaf sprigs

½ teaspoon mustard seeds

2 finely chopped small onions

2 tablespoons oil (frying and brushing)

Salt if desired

Instructions

1) Preheat the Air Fryer to 392°F.

2) Cut away the edges of the bread.

3) Peel the potatoes, and boil. Use one teaspoon of salt, and mash the potatoes.

4) In the meantime, on the stovetop use a skillet to combine the mustard seeds and one teaspoon of the oil. Add the onions when the seeds sputter, continue frying until they become translucent. Toss in the curry and turmeric.

5) Fry the mixture a few seconds, then add the salt, mashed potatoes; mix well, and let it cool.

6) Shape eight portions of the mixture into an oval shape. Set to the side.

7) Wet the bread with water, and press it into your palm to remove the excess water.

8) Place the oval potato into the bread and roll the bread completely around the potato mixture. Be sure they are completely sealed.

9) Brush the basket and the potato rolls with oil, and set to the side.

10) Set the Air Fryer timer for 12 to 13 minutes. Let them cook until crispy and browned.

Yields: Four Servings

Avocado Fries

Ingredients

1 large avocado

Pinch of black pepper and salt

¼ teaspoon paprika or cayenne pepper

¼ cup all-purpose flour

½ cup Panko breadcrumbs

1 beaten egg

¼ of a lemon

Instructions

1) Preheat the Air Fryer to 392°F.
2) Cut the avocado into eight slices.
3) Using three separate containers; add the salt, cayenne, pepper, and flour in one. Place the beaten egg in the second one and breadcrumbs in the third one.
4) Coat the avocado with the flour, egg, and breadcrumbs.
5) Put the avocado into the fryer basket and set the timer for six minutes.
6) They will be golden in color when ready to serve.

Enjoy with some Greek yogurt and honey or with a squeeze of fresh lemon juice.

Broccoli

Ingredients

2 Lbs. broccoli crowns.

2 Tablespoons olive oil

1 teaspoon kosher salt

½ teaspoon black pepper

2 teaspoons grated lemon zest

1/3 cup Kalamata olives

¼ cup shaved Parmesan cheese

Instructions

1) Remove the stems from the broccoli and cut them into 1 to 1-1/2- inch florets. Pit and cut the olives in half.
2) Over high heat, fill a medium pan with six cups of water—bring it to boiling. Toss in the florets and cook for three to four minutes. Remove and drain. Add the pepper, salt, and oil
3) Set the AF to 400°F.
4) Place the broccoli into the basket, close the drawer, and click the timer for 15 minutes. Toss/flip at seven minutes for even browning. When done, place the broccoli in the bowl.
5) Garnish with lemon zest, olives, and cheese. Enjoy immediately.

Yields: Two to Four Servings

Fact: The Kalamata olive is a native of southern Greece which is often times preserved in olive oil or wine vinegar. It is an additional 'kick' for this treat!

Buffalo Cauliflower

Ingredients

1 cup breadcrumbs

4 cups cauliflower florets

¼ cup buffalo sauce

¼ cup melted butter

For the Dip: Your favorite dressing

Instructions

1) Place the butter in a microwaveable dish; remove and whisk in the buffalo sauce.
2) Dip each of the florets in the buttery mixture; the stem does not need to have sauce. Use the stem as a handle, hold it over a cup and let the excess drip away.
3) Run the floret through the breadcrumbs to your liking. Drop them into the fryer. Cook for 14 to 17 minutes at 350°F. (The unit will not need to preheat since it is calculated in the time.)
4) You can shake the basket several times to be sure it is evenly browning. Enjoy with your favorite dip, but be sure to eat it right away because the crunchiness goes away quickly.

Note: Reheat in the oven. Don't reheat it in the microwave; it will be mushy.

Yields: Four Servings

Cheesy Potatoes

Ingredients

7 medium potatoes

½ cup grated Gruyere (semi-mature) cheese

½ cup cream

½ cup milk

1 teaspoon black pepper

½ teaspoon nutmeg

Instructions

1) Peel and slice the potatoes wafer-thin. Russet potatoes work great with this recipe.
2) Preset the Air Fryer to 400°F.
3) Blend the milk and cream; add the nutmeg pepper, and salt for seasoning.
4) Generously coat the potatoes with the mixture.
5) Put the slices in an 8 x 8 dish, pouring the rest of the mixture over the potatoes.
6) Place the dish into Air Fryer and set the timer for 25 minutes.
7) Remove the dish and sprinkle the cheese over the hot potatoes.
8) Continue cooking until the cheese is melted and browned, usually an additional ten minutes.

Yields: Serves Six

French Fried Potatoes

Ingredients

6 medium peeled potatoes

2 Tbsp. olive oil

Instructions

1) Preheat the Air Fryer to 360°F.
2) Peel and cut the potatoes into 3-inch strips x ¼-inch.
3) Soak the cut potatoes for a minimum of thirty minutes in water, and drain thoroughly. Pat them dry with a towel.
4) Coat the potatoes with the oil in a large mixing container. .
5) Drop the potatoes into the cooking basket for about thirty minutes or until they are the desired doneness.
6) Shake the basket two or three times during the cooking phase.

Note: The time may vary depending on the thickness of the potatoes.

Potatoes au Gratin

Ingredients

7 Medium peeled russet potatoes

½ cup each:

- Cream

- Milk

½ teaspoon nutmeg

1 teaspoon black pepper

½ cup semi-mature (Gruyere) grated cheese

Instructions

1) Preheat the Air Fryer to 390°F.
2) Wash and slice the potatoes wafer-thin.
3) Blend together the cream and milk—flavoring with some pepper, salt, and nutmeg.
4) Use the milk mixture to coat the potatoes.
5) Place the slices into an eight-inch baking pan/dish and pour the remainder of the milk/cream mixture on top of the potatoes.
6) Place the heat-resistant dish onto the cooking basket—setting the timer for 25 minutes.
7) Take the basket out and sprinkle with the cheese.
8) Bake ten more minutes or until browned.

Note: You can use two eggs instead of milk.

Yields: Six Servings

Homemade AF Croutons

Try these with a healthy salad:

Ingredients

Stale Bread

Butter

Optional: Olive oil

Instructions

1) Preheat the Air Fryer for about two to three minutes at 248°F. (You can always adjust the time but don't hotter than 320°F.)
2) Cube some of the old bread to the sizes you want to use for your meal. Pour in the olive oil and melted butter.
3) Put the cubed bread into the basket and cook for two to three minutes.
4) Toss and cook for an additional two to three minutes.
5) Completely cool and keep in an airtight container for no more than two days.

Portobello Mushrooms

Ingredients

1.4 Oz. cubed ham (about two slices)

4 Tbsp. extra virgin olive oil

7.05 Oz. Portobello mushrooms

2 shiitake or button mushrooms

1.8 Oz. Mozzarella cheese (shredded)

1 Tbsp. chopped garlic

Optional: Ground black pepper and salt

Instructions

1) Preheat the AF cooker at 356°F.

2) Clean, cap, and remove the stalks from the mushrooms; use a couple of paper towels to pat them dry.

3) Use 1/2 of the oil to brush the Portobello mushrooms tops and place them cap side down on a baking tray lined with aluminum foil or parchment paper.

4) Divide the mushrooms and top with cheese, garlic, the other half of mushrooms—diced, and the cubed ham.

5) Flavor with the pepper and salt. Drizzle a bit of the oil over the mushrooms.

6) Cook for about 10 minutes. Garnish with some dried or fresh parsley.

The Blooming Onion

Ingredients

4 small/medium onions

4 dollops of butter

1 Tbsp. olive oil

Instructions

1) Peel the skin from the onion and cut away the top and bottom to reveal flat ends.

2) Soak the onions in salt water for four hours to take away the harshness.

3) You'll need to cut the onion as far down as you can without severing the onion. Cut four times to make eight segments.

4) Preheat the fryer to 350°F.

5) Put the onions in the fryer and drizzle with the oil—placing a dollop of butter on each one.

6) Cook in the AF until the outside is dark, usually about thirty minutes.

Note: 4 dollops is 4 heaping tablespoons

Yields: Four Servings

Onion Rings

Ingredients

For a side dish or quick snack; purchase four ounces of frozen, battered onion rings.

Instructions

1) Preheat the Air Fryer cooker to 360°F.

2) Place the frozen onion rings in the basket for ten minutes.

3) Take them from the cooker and give them a toss.

4) Reset the timer for an additional ten minutes or more if needed.

Fat-Free Fries

Ingredients

1 to 2 sweet potatoes

1 to 2 red potatoes

Sprinkle of pepper and salt

Cooking spray

Optional: Parsley

Instructions

1) Preset the Air Fryer for 356°F.

2) Peel and cut the potatoes; place in a container of water until ready for frying.

3) Use two layers of paper towels to dry the wedges and spray them with the oil.

4) Place a single layer of fries in the basket and set the timer for ten minutes.

5) After the time is up, give the fries a shake, return to the AF for an additional eight to ten minutes.

6) Take them from the fryer and season as you wish.

Garnish with a bit of parsley.

Potato Croquets

Ingredients

7 small cubed red potatoes

1 egg yolk

2 Tablespoons all-purpose flour

½ cup grated Parmesan cheese

1 Pinch Each:

- Cayenne

- Black pepper
- Salt

For the Breading:

1 cup all-purpose flour

2 Tablespoons vegetable oil

2 beaten eggs

½ cup panko

1 Pinch of nutmeg

Instructions

1) Preset the temperature on the Air Fryer to 390°F.
2) In salted water, boil the potatoes for 15 minutes, drain, and mash. Cool completely.
3) Add the flour, cheese, and egg yolk—flavoring with nutmeg, pepper, and salt,
4) Shape the filling into golf ball size.
5) Make a crumbly mixture of the breadcrumbs and oil. Put each ball into the flour mixture, the eggs, and then the panko. Roll them into cylinder shapes.
6) Put them in the cooking basket until browned—about seven to eight minutes.

Yields: It will probably take 2 batches depending on how large you made the balls.

Potato Skin Wedges

Ingredients

6 medium russet potatoes

1 ½ tsp. paprika

½ tsp. salt

2 Tbsp. canola oil

½ tsp. black pepper

Instructions

1) Thoroughly wash the potatoes under the tap. Boil the potatoes in salted water about forty minutes.

2) Cool in the refrigerator for about thirty minutes. Quarter them when cooled.

3) Combine the paprika, pepper, salt, and oil in a mixing dish. Toss the potatoes in the mixture.

4) Place in the cooking basket with the skin side down. Cook them until golden brown; about 14 to 16 minutes.

Grilled Tomatoes AF Style

Ingredients

2 tomatoes

Cooking spray

Pepper

Herbs

Instructions

1) Preheat the fryer to 320°F.

2) Wash and cut the tomatoes into halves. Spray each of them lightly with some cooking spray and place them cut side facing upwards. Sprinkle with your favorite spices—fresh or dried—including the pepper, sage, rosemary, basil, oregano, and any others of your choice.

3) Put them into the basket for 20 minutes or until they are to the doneness you want to achieve. If they are ready to enjoy—if not—cook for a few more minutes.

This would be tasty breakfast or as a side dish.

Yields: Two Servings

Chapter 5: Air Fryer Desserts

Blackberry Apricot Crumble

Ingredients

5 ½ ounces fresh blackberries

2 tablespoons lemon juice

18 ounces fresh apricots

½ cup sugar

Pinch of salt

1 cup flour

5 tablespoons cold butter

Instructions

1) Preheat the Air Fryer to 390°F.
2) Prepare an eight-inch oven dish with a small amount of cooking oil.
3) Remove the stones, cut the apricots into cubes, and place them in a container.
4) Mix the lemon juice, blackberries, and 2 tablespoons of sugar with the apricots and mix. Place the fruit in the oven dish.
5) Combine a pinch of salt, the remainder of the sugar, and the flour in a mixing container. Add 1 tablespoon cold water and the butter; using your fingertips to make a crumbly mixture.

6) Sprinkle the crumbles over the fruit and press down.

7) Place the dish into the basket and slide it into the Air Fryer for 20 minutes. It is ready when it is cooked thoroughly, and the top is browned.

Cheesecake: Lemon Ricotta

Ingredients

1 lemon

²/³ cups (150g) sugar

2 cups (500g) ricotta

2 teaspoons vanilla essence

Instructions

1) Zest and juice the lemon.

2) Preset the Air Fryer to 320°F.

3) Mix the sugar, ricotta, 1 tablespoon lemon juice as well as the zest, and the vanilla essence—stirring until fully mixed. Blend in the cornstarch and pour into the oven dish.

4) Place the dish in the Air Fryer basket and set the timer for 25 minutes.

5) The middle should be set when the cake is complexly done.

6) Leave the cheesecake on a wire rack to fully cool.

Cherry Pie

Ingredients

2 refrigerated pre-made pie crusts

1 Can cherry pie filling (21-ounces)

1 tablespoon milk

1 egg yolk

Instructions

1) Preheat the fryer to 310°F.
2) Stab holes into the crust after placing into a pie plate. Allow the excess to hang over the edges. Place in the AF for five minutes
3) Take the basket out and set the crust on the counter. Fill it with the cherries. Remove the excess crust.
4) Cut the remainder crust into ¾-inch strips placing them as a lattice across the pie.
5) Make an egg wash with the milk and egg; brush the pie.
6) Bake for fifteen minutes.
7) Serve with the ice cream of your choice.

Yields: Eight Servings

Donut Bread Pudding

Ingredients

6 glazed donuts

4 raw egg yolks

1 ½ cups whipping cream

¼ cup sugar

¾ cup frozen sweet cherries

1 teaspoon cinnamon

½ cup semi-sweet chocolate baking chips

½ cup raisins

Instructions

1) Preheat the fryer at 310°F.

2) Combine the wet ingredients in a container and combine the rest of the ingredients and mix.

3) Pour into a baking pan and cover it with foil. Place it into the basket and set the timer for 60 minutes.

4) Chill the bread pudding well before serving.

Yields: Four Servings

Fluffy Peanut Butter Marshmallow Turnovers

Ingredients

4 defrosted sheets filo pastry

4 Tbsp. chunky peanut butter

2-ounces melted butter

4 tsp. marshmallow fluff

A Pinch of sea salt

Instructions

1) Preset the temperature of the Air Fryer to 360°F.

2) Use the melted butter to brush one sheet of the filo. Put the second sheet on top and brush it also with butter.

3) Continue the process until you have completed all four sheets.

4) Cut the layers into four (4) 12-inch x 3-inch strips.

5) Place one teaspoon of the marshmallow fluff on the underside and 1 tablespoon of the peanut butter.

6) Fold the tip over the filo strip to form a triangle, making sure the filling is completely wrapped.

7) Seal the ends with a small amount of butter. Place the completed turnovers into the AF for three to five minutes.

8) When done, they will be fluffy and golden brown.

9) Add a touch of sea salt for the sweet/salty combo.

Notes: The Filo/Phyllo pastry is a little different than regular pastry. It is tissue thin and has very little fat content. It is considered okay by some bakers and is interchange the filo with regular puff pastry for turnovers.

Yields: Four Servings

Marshmallow and Yam Hand Pies

Ingredients

1 crescent dough sheet

1 (16-ounce can) candied yams

1/2 teaspoon cinnamon

1/4 teaspoon allspice

2 tablespoons marshmallow crème

1/4 teaspoon salt

1 egg, beaten

For the Maple Glaze:

1/2 cup maple syrup

½ cup confectioners' sugar

Instructions

1) Pre-set the heat on the AF to 400°F.
2) Drain the syrup from the yams. Combine the cinnamon, salt, allspice, and yams using a fork to the blend the spices and smash the yams.
3) Put the dough sheet onto a board and cut into four equal sections.
4) Spoon the filling onto the squares and add a tablespoon of the crème.
5) Use a brush to spread the egg over the edges of the dough and place the remainder of the two pieces of dough on top of the pies.
6) Use a fork to crimp the edges and cut three slits into the top for venting.
7) Place in the Air Fryer for six minutes.
8) Make the glaze from the sugar and syrup in a small dish—slowly adding the syrup—until the sugar dissolves.

9) To serve, drizzle the glaze over the warm pies and enjoy.

Yields: Four Servings.

Orange and Pineapple Fondant

Ingredients

4.2 ounces (115) g Butter

4.2 ounces (115 g) Dark chocolate

2 medium eggs

4 tablespoons castor sugar (see note below)

2 tablespoons self-rising flour

1 medium orange (rind and juice)

Instructions

1) Grease four ramekins with a small amount of oil or cooking spray.
2) Pre-set the heat in the Air Fryer to 356°F/380°C.
3) Cut and tear apart the orange and grate the orange peel.
4) Melt the butter and chocolate in a double boiler or in a glass measuring cup over a pot of hot water. Stir until it is creamy smooth.
5) Beat and whisk in the sugar and eggs—until frothy and pale. Blend in the sugar and egg mixture along with the orange bits. Add the flour and

mix until well-blended.

6) Fill the ramekins about ¾ of the way full with the mixture. Cook in the Air Fryer for 12 minutes.

7) Take it from the fryer and let them rest for two minutes. (They will continue to cook.) Turn them out of the containers (upside down) into a serving platter. You can loosen the edges by tapping the ramekin gently with a butter knife.

8) The fondant will release from the center to provide you with a luscious center of pudding.

9) Garnish with some caramel sauce or vanilla ice cream.

Yields: Four Servings

How to Make Castor Sugar

Castor or caster sugar is simply granulated sugar that has been placed into a blender or food processor to make it a 'super-fine' sugar used for some recipes since it melts easier.

Instructions

1) Put the granulated sugar into the blender/food processor.

2) Pulse until it is a 'super-fine' texture—not powdery.

Pineapple Sticks with Yogurt Dip

Ingredients

¼ C. desiccated (moisture-free) coconut

1 C. vanilla yogurt

1 small sprig fresh mint

Instructions

1) Preheat the Air Fryer to 392°F.
2) Meanwhile, use similar shapes and sizes to cut the pineapple into sticks.
3) Dip the sticks into the coconut. Place the pineapple sticks in the basket and cook for ten minutes
4) *For the Dip*: Dice the mint into the yogurt.

Yields: Four Servings

Strawberry Cupcakes and Strawberry Icing

Ingredients

½ cup castor sugar

½ cup butter

2 medium eggs

½ cup self-rising flour

½ cup butter

½ teaspoon vanilla essence

½ cup icing sugar

1 tablespoon whipped cream

½ teaspoon pink food coloring

¼ cup fresh (blended) strawberries

Instructions

1) Set the Air Fryer temperature to 338°F/170°C.

2) Cream the sugar and butter in a large mixing container until it is creamy smooth.

3) Add the eggs one at a time along with the vanilla essence.

4) Blend in a small amount of flour at a time until all is completely mixed.

5) Pour them into ramekins about 80% of the way full. Place them in the Air Fryer for eight minutes.

6) *Make the Frosting:* Cream the butter and slowly mix in the icing sugar until creamy. Pour in the food coloring, (blended) strawberries, and whipped cream—mix well.

7) Take them out and use a piping bag to make the swirly frosting for a tasty 'pretty' cupcake every time.

Yields: Ten Servings

Chapter 6: Air Fryer Appetizers and Snacks

Cheesy Garlic Bread

Ingredients

5 round bread slices

5 teaspoons sun-dried tomato pesto

3 chopped garlic cloves

4 Tbsp. melted butter

1 cup grated Mozzarella cheese

Garnish Options:

- Chili flakes
- Chopped basil leaves
- oregano

Instructions

1) Preheat the Air Fryer to 356°F.
2) Cut the loaf of bread into 5 thick slices.
3) Add the butter, pesto, and cheese on the bread.
4) Put the slices in the preheated cooker for six to eight minutes.
5) Garnish with your choice of toppings.

Note: Round or Baguette bread was used for this recipe. It is recommended to add the finely chopped garlic cloves to the melted butter ahead of time for the best results.

Clams Oregano

Ingredients

2 dozen shucked clams

1 cup unseasoned breadcrumbs

4 tablespoons melted butter

3 clove minced garlic

1 teaspoon dried oregano

¼ cup chopped parsley

¼ cup grated Parmesan cheese

For the Pan:

- 1 cup sea salt

Instructions

1) Preheat the AF to 400°F.
2) Mix the oregano, parsley, parmesan cheese, breadcrumbs, and melted butter in a medium container.
3) Using a heaping tablespoon of the crumb mixture; add it to the exposed clams.
4) Fill the insert with the salt, place the clams inside and cook for three minutes.

5) Dress them up with a garnish of lemon wedges and fresh parsley.

Yields: Four Servings

Corn Tortilla Chips

Ingredients

8 corn Tortillas

1 Tbsp. olive oil

Salt if desired

Instructions

1) Preset the AF to 392°F.

2) Use a sharp knife to cut the tortillas.

3) Brush each tortilla with oil.

4) Air fry two batches for three minutes each. Sprinkle with a pinch of salt.

Crab Sticks

Ingredients

1 package 'DoDo' crab sticks

Cooking spray

Instructions

1) Take each of the sticks out of the package; find an edge, and unroll until flat.

2) Tear the sheets into 1/3 widths.

3) Place them on a plate and coat them with cooking spray.

4) Cook them in the AF for 10 minutes.

5) *Note*: If you shred the crab meat; you can cut the time in half, but they will also easily fall through the holes in the basket.

Garlic Knots

Ingredients

Marinara sauce

1 teaspoon sea salt

1 Lb. frozen pizza crust dough

1 tablespoon each:

- Garlic powder
- Grated Parmesan cheese
- Fresh chopped parsley

Instructions

1) Preheat the Air Fryer to 360°F.

2) Roll out the dough until is about 1 ½ to 2-inches thick. Slice it approximately ¾-inches apart—lengthwise.

3) Roll the dough and make it into knots.

4) Add the cheese, oil, and spices in a bowl, and roll each knot in the mixture before placing it into the fry basket.

5) Set the timer for 12 minutes; flipping halfway through the cooking process (six minutes).

Serve with a dish of marinara sauce.

Yields: Four Servings

Kale Chips

Ingredients

1 Tbsp. olive oil

1 head of kale

1 tsp. Soya sauce

Instructions

1) De-stem the kale and tear it into 1 1/2 –inch pieces.
2) Rinse in cold water and thoroughly dry using some paper towels.
3) Toss the kale with the soya sauce and oil.
4) Set the Air Fryer for 200°F for two to three minutes; toss when half cooked.

Meatballs for the Party

Ingredients

2 ½ Tablespoons Worcestershire sauce

1 pound ground beef

1 Tablespoon Tabasco

¾ cup tomato ketchup

1 Tablespoon lemon juice

¼ cup vinegar

½ teaspoon dry mustard

½ cup brown sugar

3 crushed gingersnaps

Instructions

1) Combine all of the seasonings in a large mixing container—blending well.

2) Mix the beef and continue churning the ingredients.

3) Make the balls and put them in the fryer. Cook on 375°F for 15 minutes.

4) Place them on the toothpicks before serving.

Note: They are ready when the center is done, and they are crispy.

Yields: 24 Servings

Feta Triangles

Ingredients

4 ounces feta cheese

1 egg yolk

2 tablespoons finely chopped flat-leafed parsley

2 sheets frozen (defrosted) filo pastry

1 finely chopped scallion

2 tablespoons olive oil

Ground black pepper

Instructions

1) Pre-set the heat in the Air Fryer to 390°F.

2) Whisk the egg and blend in the scallion, feta, and parsley.

3) Cut the dough into three strips.

4) Place a heaping teaspoon of the feta mix underneath the pastry strip.

5) Fold the tip to form a triangle as you work your way around the strip.

6) Use a small amount of oil and brush each of the triangles before placing them in the cooker basket cooking them for three minutes.

7) Lower the heat to 360°F, and continue cooking for an additional two minutes.

Yields: Five Servings

Mozzarella Sticks

Ingredients

2 eggs

1 pound or block Mozzarella cheese

1 cup plain breadcrumbs

¼ cup white flour

3 tablespoons nonfat milk

Instructions

1) Preheat the fryer to 400°F.

2) Slice the cheese into ½-inch x 3-inch sticks.

3) Whisk the milk and egg together in one bowl, with the oil and bread crumbs in individual dishes as well.

4) Dredge the sliced cheese through the oil, egg, and breadcrumbs.

5) Place the sticks on bread tin and put them in the freezer compartment for about an hour or two.

6) Place them in small increments (don't overcrowd) into the AF basket.

7) Cook for 12 minutes.

Yields: Four Servings

Mini Quiche Wedges

Ingredients

1 (3 ½ ounces or 100 g) Frozen or ready-made pizza crust

1 egg

(1.4 ounces or 40 g) Grated cheese

½ tablespoon oil

3 tablespoons whipping cream

Fresh ground pepper

2 small pie molds

Instructions

1) Pre-set the heat on the Air Fryer to 392°F/200°C.

2) Use a bit of cooking spray to grease the molds. Line them with the dough pressing down around the edges.

3) Whisk the cheese, cream, and egg flavoring with some pepper and salt to taste. Empty the mixture into the molds.

4) Put the mold into the basket and set the timer for 12 minutes. Bake the second one the same way.

5) Take them from the molds and slice each of the quiche into six wedges.

6) You can serve at room temperature or warm.

Try these Variations:

Ingredients for Mushroom Slices

4.4 ounces or 125 g sliced mushrooms

1 teaspoon paprika

1 crushed clove of garlic

OR

Ingredients Ham and Broccoli

1.8 ounces or 50 g small broccoli florets and ham

Instructions for Ham and Broccoli

Boil the florets until tender.

Divide between each of the quiches.

Yields: Nine Servings

Spicy Pumpkin Patch Cannoli Treats for Halloween

Ingredients

4 tablespoons melted butter

8 large flour tortillas

1 cup sugar

½ cup orange sanding sugar

2 pounds whole milk ricotta

1 tablespoon ground cinnamon

2/3 cup confectioners' sugar

1 ½ cup pumpkin pie mix

½ cup mini chocolate chips

Instructions

1) Preheat the Air Fryer for three minutes at 400°F.
2) Use a pumpkin cookie cutter to make the tortillas.
3) Brush one side of the cutouts with the butter and sprinkle them with the orange sanding sugar.
4) Mix the cinnamon a regular sugar in a small dish; sprinkle over the cookies.
5) Bake the treats in batches until crispy (about three minutes).
6) Use wire racks for cooling.
7) Make the dip by using a large bowl and combining the cinnamon sugar, pumpkin pie, mix, and ricotta in a large mixing dish. Stir well.
8) Be creative and place the dip in a shallow serving platter.
9) Place the crisps into the dip to make a pumpkin patch and decorate with the chips.

Yields: Four Servings

Sweet Potato Chips

Ingredients

2 Large Sweet potatoes

1 Tbsp. olive oil

Instructions

1) Pre-set the heat in the Air Fryer to 350°F.
2) Peel and slice the potatoes into chips. It is best to slice them into the same sizes so then will cook evenly.
3) Place the potatoes into a resealable baggie and add the oil. Shake the potatoes to coat them completely.
4) Pour the sweet potatoes into the Air Fryer and cook for approximately fifteen minutes, depending on the thickness.

Conclusion

Thank for viewing your personal copy of the *Air Fryer Cookbook Mastery: Your Ultimate Air Fryer Recipe Book For Quick, Easy, And Healthy Foods*. Let's hope it was informative and provided you with all of the valuable information you need to achieve your goals whether you are seeking a way to lose weight or any just want to live a healthier lifestyle. Life cannot be much simpler than this.

The next step is to decide which recipe you want to test out first. Do you remember these?

- Banana Fritters
- Coconut Shrimp
- Spicy Rolled Meat
- Orange and Chocolate Fondant
- Bread Rolls with Potato Stuffing

Does any of that strike your fancy for this evening?

Finally, if you found this book useful in any way; a review on Amazon is always appreciated!

VIP Subscriber List

Hi Dear Reader, this is Diana! If you like my book and you want to receive the latest tips and tricks on cooking, weight-loss, cookbook recipes and more, do subscribe to my mailing list in the link here! I will then be able to send you the most up-to-date information about my upcoming books and promotions as well! Thank you for supporting my work and happy reading!

Subscriber Form

http://bit.do/dianawatson

Index

Chapter 2: Breakfast Recipes

- Apple Dumplings
- Banana Fritters
- French Toast Sticks
- Bacon and Eggs
- Cheesy Mushroom, Ham, and Egg
- Scrambled Eggs
- Air Fryer Spinach Frittata
- Bacon Wrapped Tater Tots
- Buttermilk Biscuits
- Vegan Mini Bacon Wrapped Burritos

Chapter 3: Lunch Recipes

- Grilled Cheese Sandwich
- Cheeseburger Mini Sliders
- Pigs In A Blanket

Chicken

- AF Chicken 'Fried'

- AF Buffalo Chicken Wings
- Chinese Chicken Wings
- Country Style Chicken Tenders
- Chicken Pot Pie
- Tarragon Chicken

Beef

- Beef Roll Ups
- Air Fried Ravioli
- Roasted Veggie Pasta Salad

Chapter 4: Dinner Recipes

Chicken and Turkey Recipes

- Lemon Rosemary Chicken
- Jamaican Chicken Meatballs
- Roast Turkey Breast

- Spicy Rolled Meat

Fish and Seafood

- Salmon Patties

- Dill Salmon

- Halibut Steak With a Teriyaki Glazed Sauce

- Cajun Shrimp

- Coconut Shrimp

Beef

- Rib Steak

- Stromboli

- Roasted Rack of Lamb with a Macadamia Crust

- Crispy Tofu

Sides

- Bread Rolls with Potato Stuffing

- Avocado Fries

- Broccoli

- Buffalo Cauliflower

- Cheesy Potatoes

- French Fried Potatoes

- Potatoes au Gratin

- Homemade AF Croutons

- Portobello Mushrooms

- The Blooming Onion

- Onion Rings

- Fat-Free Fries

- Potato Croquets

- Potato Skin Wedges

- Grilled Tomatoes AF Style

Chapter 5: Air Fryer Desserts

- Blackberry Apricot Crumble

- Cheesecake: Lemon Ricotta

- Cherry Pie

- Donut Bread Pudding

- Fluffy Peanut Butter Marshmallow Turnovers

- Marshmallow and Yam Hand Pies

- Orange and Chocolate Fondant

- Pineapple Sticks with Yogurt Dip

Chapter 6: Air Fryer Appetizers and Snacks

- Cheesy Garlic Bread

- Clams Oregano

- Corn Tortilla Chips

- Crab Sticks

- Garlic Knots

- Kale Chips

- Meatballs for the Party

- Feta Triangles

- Mozzarella Sticks

- Mini Quiche Wedges

- Spicy Pumpkin Patch Cannoli Treats for Halloween

- Sweet Potato Chips